On-Site Management of Scuba Diving and Boating Emergencies

Best Publishing Company

On-Site Management of Scuba Diving and Boating Emergencies

Wesley Y. Yapor, M.D.

Illustrations by David Halek

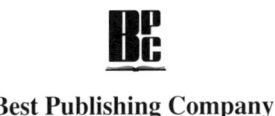

Best Publishing Company

Illustrations by David Halek
Edited by Jim Joiner
Design by Rudy Ramos and Vanessa Palacio

Copyright © 2002 by Best Publishing Company

All Rights Reserved

No part of this book may be reproduced, stored in a retrieval system, or transmitted in any form or by any means; electronic, mechanical, photocopying, microfilming, recording, or otherwise; without the permission of the publisher, except by a reviewer who may quote brief passages in a review with appropriate credit.

ISBN: 0-930536-02-X
Library of Congress Catalog Number: 2001097544

Best Publishing Company
2355 North Steves Boulevard
P.O. Box 30100
Flagstaff, AZ 86003-0100 USA
Tele: 928.527.1055
Email: divebooks@bestpub.com
website: www.bestpub.com

Dedication

This book is dedicated to the four most important people in my life, my children: Myles Prescott, Lance Nathaniel, Danielle Yvonne, and Austin Conrad. They have been and continue to be a source of endless joy and wonderful inspiration to me. Scuba diving, boating, and traveling with them has raised my awareness of safety to new heights and this has been a strong motivation for me in the preparation of this book. May they never need to use it but always have it handy.

Introduction

The scuba diver is vulnerable not only to the hazards of a swimmer, but also to those of a boater, a traveler, and to an explorer that transgresses beyond the normal boundaries of our intended environment. A wide variety of injuries, exposures, diseases, mechanical failures, and accidents may be encountered. The key to a smooth diving trip or excursion is prevention and safety. Should a problem arise, preparedness with the necessary tools and well thought out contingency plans are required to offer appropriate assistance and limit or reverse injury or damage. The capability to recognize that a problem exists and the ability to identify the type of problem and its cause will permit the individual to initiate proper treatment, action, or repair.

This book is meant to be a blueprint with which to understand and identify diving and boating medical conditions, an inventory of the proper tools and equipment for treatment, and a guide to know when and how to use them. A basic understanding of human anatomy (how the body is put together) and physiology (how the body works) is needed in order to evaluate an injured or ill person and recognize normal from abnormal. Identification and localization of the problem are essential and are the initial goals of an evaluation. The next determination is whether treatment or stabilization is to be the second goal. This decision will dictate whether to manage injuries or conditions on-site or to activate the Emergency Medical System (EMS) or Coast Guard while stabilization of the victim is attempted. Treatment rendered to an injured or ill diver must be directed toward a specific diagnosis. Therapy should never be given at random or in a shotgun-type manner. Serious consideration is to be given to the potential deleterious side effects any type of intervention may cause.

Although identifying an emergency immediately helps improve the likelihood of a good outcome it will not guarantee a good outcome. Not all rescue attempts are successful and the rescuer needs to keep in mind the possible feelings of second-guessing oneself after the fact. Feelings of guilt or decreased self-confidence are common. Hindsight can hound the conscience of a rescuer. The heightened tension and the speed of events during an emergency allow for only spontaneous reactions. Rescuers must realize that their efforts only improve the likelihood of a good outcome but do not guarantee it.

Scuba diving exposes the human body to a variety of anatomical, physiological, and psychological stresses. This subaquatic adventure may also lead to a number of hazards that range from losing one's way to vulnerability to hostile species. Without the proper gear one may also overstay one's visit or suffer from equipment malfunction. Scuba-related emergencies, medical conditions, and equipment problems are discussed and contingency protocols are described for managing them.

Boating is a fundamental part of diving and requires planning and preparation for a smooth excursion. A vast array of mechanical, weather, and water-related problems may be encountered that demand quick and specific action to avoid or limit damage. A wide range of injuries and medical conditions can be associated with boating as well. The more commonly encountered boating adversities are reviewed and the suggested action is delineated for achieving the optimal outcome.

Diving requires travel, whether to the nearby seashore or lake, or to an exotic destination. Travelers are at risk from a diversity of sources from the moment they leave the security of their home. The naive tourist may fall prey to crafty and well-seasoned crooks and may be in danger of loosing all possessions or worse. Travels abroad may also lead the unsuspecting wayfarer into regions that are endemic with opportunistic diseases or parasites. Understanding the dangers and the recommended precautions may help avoid a regretful experience. Should one become victimized the proper steps or actions may prevent a bad scenario from getting worse. The more likely travel-related problems are discussed and recommendations presented to avoid or cope with them.

Table of Contents

Dedication	V
Introduction	VII
List of Tables	XVII
List of Figures	XVIII
About the Author	XXI
About the Illustrator	XXIII

Chapter One—EQUIPMENT 1
   First Aid Kit 2
   Floats/Buoys 12
   Vessel Electronics 15
   Vessel Equipment 17
   Essential Diving Gear 20
   Boating and Diving Accessories 22
      Boating Accessories 22
      Diving Accessories 22

Chapter Two—MEDICAL EXAMINATION 27
   Physical Examination 28
      Vital Signs 28
         • Respirations 29
         • Heart Rate and Blood Pressure 29
         • Temperature 31
      Musculoskeletal System 32
         • Extremities 32
         • Head 33
         • Spine 34
      Neurological Survey 34
         • Mental Status 35

- Cranial Nerves...36
- Motor 38
- Sensation 39
- Cerebellar Function 40

Chapter Three—MEDICAL MANAGEMENT 41
Cardiopulmonary Resuscitation...41
    Airway Obstruction 45
    Cricothyroidotomy 47
    Pneumothorax and Hemothorax 49
Burns 52
    Classification 52
        - Sunburn 54
        - Fire Burns..54
        - Hot Liquids 55
        - Chemical Burns 55
        - Electrical Burns 56
        - Rope or Friction Burns....................................57
Hypothermia 57
Hyperthermia 58
    Heat Exhaustion 59
    Heat Stroke 59
Sea Sickness 60
Fractures..62
    Skull Fractures..62
    Spine Fractures...64
    Extremity Fractures 68
Concussion 69
    Coma vs. Concussion 69
Convulsions 70
Amputation 72
Hemorrhage...73
Drowning 76
Crush Injury 78
    Chest 78
    Abdominal 79

  Head 80
  Extremity 80
 Penetrating Injury 81
  Chest 82
  Abdominal 82
  Head 83
  Extremity 85
 Heart Attack 86
 Stroke...87
 Shock..88
  • Hypovolemic Shock 89
  • Anaphylactic, Septic, and Toxic Shock........................90
  • Cardiogenic Shock 91
  • Neurogenic Shock 92
 Documentation 92

Chapter Four—UNDERWATER EMERGENCIES 97
 Fatigue..98
 Panic 99
 Nitrogen Induced Problems..101
  Nitrogen Narcosis 101
  Decompression Sickness..101
 Barotrauma 103
  Ears and Sinuses...104
  Chest Cavity 105
 Lipoid Pneumonia 106
 Carbon Monoxide Poisoning..107
 Oxygen Toxicity 108
 Unconscious Diver 110
 Entanglement and Entrapment 112
 Buddy Separation/Lost Diver..115
  Buddy Separation..115
  Lost Diver...118
  Search Patterns 119
 Equipment Failure 122
  Tank..122

  BCD 123
  Weights 125
  Regulator 128
  Fins... 128
  Mask 129
  Gauges 130
 Marine Organism Attacks and Poisonings............................. 131
  Jellyfish and Coral 131
  Cone Shells... 133
  Stinging Sponges 134
  Bristle Worms 134
  Marine Snakes 135
  Sharks 135
  Crocodilians 138
  Moray Eels 139
  Barracuda 140
  Sea Urchins and Other Spiny Fish 140

Chapter Five—SURFACE EMERGENCIES 143
 Signs of Trouble 143
 Dive Entrance 144
 Boat Injuries 145
 Lost at Sea 148
 Fatigue... 153
 Panic 154
 Towing... 155
 Rescue Breathing.. 158
 Exit with a Victim 161

Chapter Six—BOATING EMERGENCIES................................ 169
 Lightning 169
 Lost at Sea 171
 Taking on Water... 177
 Collision 180
 Abandoning Ship 181
 Man Overboard 184

Fire 187
    Type A-Wood or Cloth 188
    Type B-Liquids 189
    Type C-Electrical 190
    Type D-Metals 190
    Vessel Inspection and Dewatering 191
Vessel Aground 192
Dragging Anchor 195
Power Failure 199
    Engine Failure 199
    Electrical Failure 200
Bad Weather and Rough Water 201

Chapter Seven—TRAVEL-RELATED CONDITIONS 205
Air Travel 206
    Burglary 206
    Conditions Encountered in Flight 207
        • Decompression Illness 207
        • Deep Vein Thrombosis and Pulmonary Embolus 208
        • Respiratory Infections 209
        • Turbulence 210
        • Jetlag 213
Parasites 214
    Class Insecta 216
        • Lice 216
        • Bedbugs 216
        • Fleas 217
        • Sandflies 217
        • Tsetse Flies 217
        • Ticks 218
        • Mites 218
        • Mosquitoes 219
        • Blackflies and Buffalo Gnats 219
    Class Hirudinea 220
        • Leaches 220
    Class Trematoda 221

- Fluke Worms 221
- Class Cestoidea 221
  - Pork Tapeworm 222
  - Beef Tapeworm 223
- Phylum Protozoa 223
  - Amoebas 224
- Phylum Nematoda 225
  - Threadworm 225
  - Hookworm 226
  - Roundworm 226
  - Pinworm 226
  - Whipworm 227
- Microbial Diseases 228
  - Cholera 228
  - Creutzfeldt-Jakob Disease 229
  - Salmonella 230
  - Shigella 230
  - Tuberculosis 231
  - Tinea Cruris and Tinea Pedis 233
  - Hepatitis 233
  - Dengue 235
  - Staphylococcus 235
- Lost or Stolen Credit Card or Money 236
- Assaults 238
- Motor Vehicle Precautions 242
  - Imprisonment 244

Appendix I
Example of Emergency Procedures—Check Lists 247

Appendix II
Example of Emergency Action Plan 253

Index 255

List of Tables

Table	1	First Aid Kit	11
Table	2	Floats/Buoys	14
Table	3	Vessel Electronics	16
Table	4	Vessel Equipment	19
Table	5	Essential Dive Equipment	21
Table	6	Diving and Boating Accessories	25
Table	7	Glasgow Coma Scale	36
Table	8	Cranial Nerve Function	37
Table	9	Documentation	95
Table	10	World Time Zone Chart	175
Table	11	Apparent Time Conversion Chart	176

List of Figures

Figure	1	Location of Pulses	31
Figure	2	One-Person CPR	43
Figure	3	One-Person Chest Compressions	43
Figure	4	Two-Person CPR	44
Figure	5	Heimlich Maneuver	45
Figure	6	Abdominal Thrust	46
Figure	7	Front View of Trachea	48
Figure	8	Location of Cricothyroid Membrane	48
Figure	9	Inserting Artificial Airway	48
Figure	10	Location of Needle Insertion for Pneumothorax	50
Figure	11	Insertion of Needle for Pneumothorax	51
Figure	12	Needle with Flap Valve	51
Figure	13	Percent of Body Surface Area/Burns	53
Figure	14	Three-Quarter Prone Position	66
Figure	15	Single-Rescuer Carrying Spine Victim	67
Figure	16	Two-Rescuers Carrying Spine Victim	67
Figure	17	Five-Rescuers Carrying Spine Victim	67
Figure	18	Application of Tourniquet	73
Figure	19	Shock Victim Position	90
Figure	20	Shock Victim with Spine Injury	92
Figure	21	Ascent with Unconscious Diver	112
Figure	22	Expanding Square Search	120
Figure	23	Reciprocal "U" Search	120
Figure	24	Expanding Circle Search	121
Figure	25	Shoreline Search	121
Figure	26	Swimming Down to Mooring Line	126
Figure	27	Spread Eagle in Uncontrolled Ascent	127
Figure	28	Inverted Ascent	127
Figure	29	Portuguese Man O' War	132
Figure	30	Blade Fire Coral	132

Figure	31	Cone Shell	133
Figure	32	Stinging Sponge	134
Figure	33	Bristle Worm	134
Figure	34	Hammerhead Shark	135
Figure	35	Banded Sea Snake	136
Figure	36	Yellow-Bellied Sea Snake	136
Figure	37	Reef Shark	137
Figure	38	Crocodilian	138
Figure	39	Barracuda	140
Figure	40	Sea Urchin	140
Figure	41	Rock Fish	141
Figure	42	Tucked Position	149
Figure	43	Group Huddle	149
Figure	44	Swimming to Shore with Current	150
Figure	45	Swimming to Shore Behind Island	150
Figure	46	Waving Sausage Buoy at Boat	151
Figure	47	Shining Light at Boat at Peak of Wave	152
Figure	48	Shining Light at Buoy at Trough of Wave	152
Figure	49	Tank Straddle Tow	157
Figure	50	Do-Si-Do Tow	157
Figure	51	Tank Valve Tow	157
Figure	52	Foot-Shoulder Tow	158
Figure	53	In-water Mouth-to-Mouth Rescue Breathing	160
Figure	54	In-water Mouth-to-Mask Rescue Breathing	160
Figure	55	In-water Mouth-to-Snorkel Rescue Breathing	161
Figure	56	Two-Rescuer Exit	162
Figure	57	Fireman Carry	163
Figure	58	Cradle or Arm Carry	163
Figure	59	Packstrap Carry	163
Figure	60	Saddleback Carry	163
Figure	61	Hand Pull Exit	164
Figure	62	Exit on Pier with Victim	165
Figure	63	Exit on Pier with Victim	165
Figure	64	Exit on Pier with Victim	165
Figure	65	Exit on Pier with Victim	165
Figure	66	Lifting Victim with Rope	166

Figure	67	Exit on Ladder with Victim 167
Figure	68	Lifting Victim with Tarp 168
Figure	69	Lifting Victim with Tarp 168
Figure	70	Latitude Nomogram 174
Figure	71	Covering Hole in Hull with Tarp 179
Figure	72	Extinguishing Type A Fire 189
Figure	73	Extinguishing Type B Fire 190
Figure	74	Banking Foam Off Wall 191
Figure	75	Lifting Bow to Free Vessel Aground 193
Figure	76	Using Anchor to Free Vessel Aground 194
Figure	77	Shifting Cargo to Free Vessel Aground 195
Figure	78	Change in Landmarks Bearing to Monitor Anchor ..196
Figure	79	Monitoring Anchor Drag with Landmarks 197
Figure	80	Monitoring Anchor Drag with Radar Ranges 198
Figure	81	Monitoring Anchor Drag with Drift Lead 199
Figure	82	Stabilizing Victim in Airplane Seat 211
Figure	83	Stabilizing Spine Victim in Airplane 212
Figure	84	Lice 216
Figure	85	Bed Bug 216
Figure	86	Flea 217
Figure	87	Sand Fly 217
Figure	88	Tsetse Fly 217
Figure	89	Tick 218
Figure	90	Mite 218
Figure	91	Mosquito 219
Figure	92	Black Fly 219
Figure	93	Leech 220
Figure	94	Fluke Worm 221
Figure	95	Tape Worm 222
Figure	96	Threadworm 225
Figure	97	Hookworm 226
Figure	98	Roundworm 226
Figure	99	Pinworm 227
Figure	100	Whipworm 227

About the Author

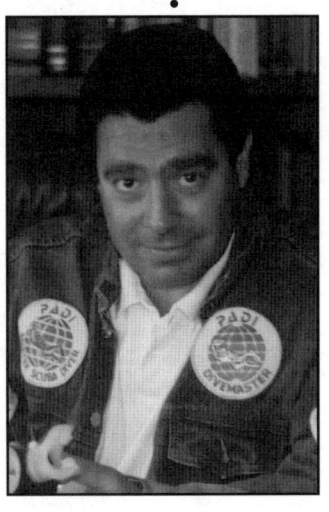

Wesley Yamil Yapor, M.D. is a PADI and NAUI certified scuba diver. His certifications include many specialties such as Rescue Diver, Master Scuba Diver, and Dive-Master. He is a member of the United States Merchant Marine, a U.S. Coast Guard licensed Master Captain for charter vessels under 50 gross tons, and licensed as a marine tow assistant. Dr. Yapor is the founder of "Elite Diving Charters" located at Waukegan Harbor, just north of Chicago. This scuba diving charter establishment is dedicated toward the safest diving in the most luxurious ambiance possible.

Dr. Yapor is a native Chicagoan and is a board-certified, assistant professor in Neurosurgery practicing and teaching in the Chicago area since 1989. His medical publications can be found in Neurosurgery, the Journal of Neurosurgery, Neurological Surgery, and the Journal of Stroke and Cerebrovascular Disease. He is the author of *Essentials of Diving Safety*, a comprehensive book on diving and boating preparedness published in the year 2000 by Best Publishing Company.

Dr. Yapor participates in emergency room coverage, which includes trauma centers. He frequently must coordinate his care of patients with a multitude of other medical specialties to optimize patient outcomes. His years of experience in medicine and boating are reflected in this excellent guide for managing diving and boating emergencies.

About the Illustrator

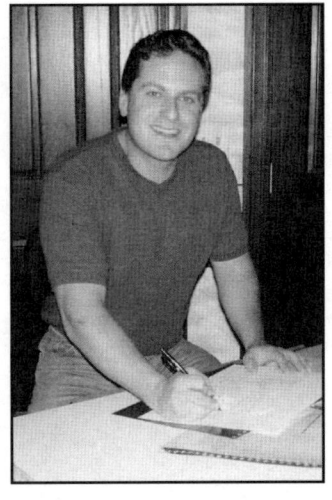

David Halek is a thirty-year-old native of Chicago, Illinois. He attended the University of Illinois at Champaign, Urbana. Later he went on to complete apprentice training with the Chicago Journeymen Plumbers Local 130 and is currently employed as a licensed plumber.

David's passion for art began as a child through comic book classics, such as Superman, which he would try to duplicate by tracing. As time went by, his imagination grew as well as his skill. David is a self-taught artist who briefly studied at the American Academy of Art. Since then David has practiced as a commissioned artist.

When he is not pursuing his love for art, David enjoys helping his wife, Lisa, care for their infant daughter, Samantha.

CHAPTER ONE
Equipment

Preparedness with the proper equipment will arm the diver and boater with the tools necessary to manage the majority of diving and boating emergencies. It would be impossible to always have all the tools needed to handle every emergency that is within the realm of possibility. The goal is to have a reasonable collection of instruments that will either manage or stabilize the most likely adverse events that may be encountered. The supply of equipment may be divided into what is needed for medical emergencies, boating adversities, and mechanical predicaments. Some of the gear may be used to prevent a predicament or to rectify a problem, and other instruments are intended for obtaining help or backup.

As important as having the proper tools and medications one must also consider the ability to call for help and activate the Emergency Medical System (EMS) or the U.S. Coast Guard in the local area in the event of an emergency. Every dive trip must have an established method of calling for help whether it be a ship to shore radio or by a portable or public phone on shore dives. All pertinent phone numbers to emergency services and the radio frequencies monitored by the authorities must be listed on an Emergency Action Plan (EAP) Sheet, (see appendix 2). This EAP sheet ought to be accessible and its location known to each diver. All those on the dive must also know the location and procedures for use of the radio or phone. Having an "Emergency Procedures" checklist (See Appendix 1) is important and required on many vessels so that crew and passengers may refer to it in case of fire, collision, taking on water, man overboard, injury, and other adverse circumstances. This checklist should include the location of the life vests, fire extinguishers, the first aid kit, the emergency leak repair kit, flares, and any other pertinent items required during an emergency. The "Emergency Procedures" checklist may also include instructions on the use of the marine radio, and protocols for calling for help. The vessel's specifications including the boat's call numbers may be included for convenient reference. The Emergency Action Plan that contains the numbers of all the local EMS personnel and local harbors may be included as part of the "Emergency Procedures" checklist.

The following inventory of equipment is divided up into "Kits" or "stores of apparatus" and intended to prepare the diver or boater for the event a misadventure is encountered.

First Aid Kit

All dive excursions need a first aid kit with the equipment that may be useful during the most commonly encountered diving and boating injuries and conditions. Management of any medical emergency requires a few basic items. Most of these items are meant to manage minor problems or to stabilize a major problem until definitive care is delivered at a medical facility. There are first aid kits available through DAN (Divers Alert Network) and other organizations that are fairly well equipped for most emergencies.

Although the list of items suggested seems rather extensive, all these items excluding the oxygen tank and blanket can fit in a container the size of a shoebox and can easily fit into a dive bag.

Although an emergency medical kit will be limited and unable to handle all possible scenarios that might occur at a dive site, it can be equipped to *temporize* until definitive help can arrive if serious injury were to occur. It is best if an emergency medical kit has a manual (such as this one) and/or slates that describe the treatments for the more common injuries or conditions. Using an emergency slate or manual to follow recommended protocols and carefully documenting the event, not only assures that the victim will receive proper care but the rescuers will have proof that they followed accepted norms for the circumstances at hand. A detailed and complete record of what was done and when it was administered will help medical personnel and protect the rescuers in the future if questions are raised or an investigation is conducted.

Two common life-threatening conditions divers experience are decompression injuries and decompression sickness. Delivery of high oxygen concentrations is the best first aid a diver can receive in the field. For this reason all dive boats should have an oxygen tank aboard. The size of the tank must be appropriate for the required time needed to get emergency help to the patient. Thirty minutes of oxygen, for example is inadequate for a one-hour cruise. The oxygen delivery valves (demand-valve) help to diminish oxygen loss and prolong the tank's usefulness. The crew must be familiar with the indications to begin oxygen therapy as well as the use of the mask and valve. The delivery of oxygen to a diver suffering from near drowning, smoke inhalation, decompression sickness, or a decompression injury should begin immediately and continue until the victim is in the hands of the Emergency Medical System. Oxygen is also needed for the diver who has omitted a required decompression that could not be completed because of oversight or lack of air. The diver who ascends too quickly, omits a safety stop, or aspirates water (inhaled water) and has a significant choking and coughing spell might also benefit from oxygen therapy depending upon the circumstances.

Before going on a dive trip, be sure the medication in the emergency medical kit has not expired. This may be done several days before the intended trip to ensure sufficient time to restock the medication list. The medication most commonly used while on a boat dive is the anti-emetic (anti-nausea drugs). It is suggested that anti-emetics are more effective if they are taken in combination with other anti-emetics that work on different modes of action. One should consult one's physician about these medications before using any of them either singly or in combination. If one does have a medication that one has taken safely, it is more effective if administered about one half-hour before boarding a boat. If the Scopalamine patches are used the boater should be careful to wash their hands after handling the patch and avoid touching the area around the eye. If the medication comes in contact with the eye it will cause dilatation of the pupil and result in blurred vision until the medication wears off.

Aspirin is a recommended pain reliever to have on hand. If an injury results in bleeding, or if internal bleeding is suspected, avoid the use of aspirin as it will inhibit the function of platelets that are essential for clotting to occur. Aspirin is recommended for victims if a heart attack is suspected. Ibuprofen or acetaminophen are alternative pain medication for minor injuries. Isopropyl alcohol, peroxide, ammonia, and Betadine™ solution are excellent antiseptics and should be part of a complete kit. In areas where there may be jellyfish or coral, a bottle of vinegar may be included in the first aid kit to deactivate the nematocysts of jellyfish stings and coral. Saline eyewash may be useful for a variety of eye injuries or contaminations. Benadryl™ is an antihistamine that may be appropriate for a multitude of allergic reactions or rashes due to chemical or material exposures or toxins. A nasal decongestant spray or oral decongestants may be useful for divers with difficulty clearing their ears or sinuses. These agents need to be used carefully to prevent the medication from wearing off and producing a reverse squeeze upon ascent. Other medication such as local anesthetics, epinephrine, antibiotics, anti-venom, intravenous saline solution, and others would be appropriate for medically trained individuals and part of a more advanced life support setup. Having some ice is advisable to be used for a variety of injuries.

Local anesthetic is a very useful drug to have. There are creams and sprays that will deliver local anesthesia to an area without the need for an injection. The advantage of the injected anesthetic is that it delivers a much more effective anesthetic and is almost immediate in its onset. The sprays and creams take a significant period of time to work and produce less than total anesthesia. Allergies could be a complicating factor when delivering an anesthetic. A history of allergies must be pursued before giving a victim an anesthetic. The proper application of an injected local anesthetic requires knowledge of body anatomy and the ability to be sure one does not inject the anesthetic directly into a blood vessel or nerve. The application of the anesthetic into the proper tissue plane is important as well and this is why only an individual trained in its use should perform the injection of a local anesthetic.

Sunscreens can be a trip saver. Nothing is more easily prevented than sunburn. Having sunscreen with a high SPF (Sun Protection Factor) rating, 15 or greater, is recommended. Other creams and ointments to keep handy would be burn creams, antibiotic cream, a steroid cream (cortisone), anesthetic cream (pain reliever), moisturizer, lip balm, and Vaseline™ petroleum.

Petroleum ointment is important to apply to injuries where an area may be denuded of healthy skin. Wounds such as burns, avulsions, multiple puncture wounds, blistering reactions, and others may benefit from application of an ointment (oil-based) to prevent loss of fluid from the victim. Petroleum ointment can also be used to seal in another medication. If treating a burn victim one can first cool the tissues with cold water. Then apply an anesthetic cream to decrease the pain and cover the cream with the petroleum ointment to prevent water loss and lock in the anesthetic. Covering the treated area with a clear plastic wrap will keep the medication from being absorbed by the dressing. This is then dressed with sterile gauze. The same can be done with a steroid cream in an area with an allergic reaction, a moisturizing cream on an area parched by the sun (lips), a burn cream for superficial or deep burns, etc.

The recommended bandages include small, medium, and large adhesive bandages, gauze in folded squares and in rolled lengths, cotton swabs, and eye pads or dressings. Bandage tape, steri-strip wound closure strips, Ace wraps™, ankle braces, splints, a blanket, tincture of benzoin, and a tourniquet or string is important as well. Ace wraps™ can be used for a variety of purposes. They can be used to form slings or to add support to an unstable or injured joint. A temporary cast can be made of newspaper, magazines, and sticks or poles of the appropriate length. These temporary casts can be wrapped with the Ace wraps™ for support. The tightness of the wrap should be carefully monitored to be sure that vascular compression does not reduce or eliminate blood flow to an extremity. An Ace wrap™ is never to be used around the neck to avoid compression on the trachea, carotid arteries, or jugular veins. Upon occasion a pressure dressing is called for if significant bleeding is encountered from an area. Direct pressure is the best solution to control the bleeding but a tight wrap may be needed to act as a tourniquet as a last resort.

Gauze is useful to protect a wound and to form surface area for blood to coagulate in order to stop bleeding. If an open wound is being packed to stop bleeding, the gauze can be made more effective if unfolded and packed with moderate pressure. Counting the number of gauze pieces that are placed in the wound is important. Keeping track of materials used and placed in or on a victim must be forwarded to healthcare personnel. Gauze soaked in peroxide is frequently used in hospitals to stop bleeding. Peroxide or Betadine™ on gauze may be used to sterilize a wound. Alcohol is avoided due to the severe pain it causes. Peroxide causes minimal if any discomfort. Wounds that are packed with gauze may be covered with folded dry gauze squares and secured with tape, or the wound is then wrapped with long gauze rolls or Ace wraps™. Gauze is the preferred material to be used to clean a superficial wound with either peroxide or alcohol. Be careful never to allow either peroxide or alcohol to enter the eyes. Eye contamination may occur easily when caring for a wound on the face or head. Cotton balls are not the preferred material to pack wounds and should be avoided in large open wounds. They may be difficult to find and may be a source of future problems if left in the wound. They are good for covering the ear if drops are placed and to care for superficial wounds or for eye care. They are good to stop bleeding from puncture sites but are not to be pushed into the puncture tract.

An assortment of different sized bandages is commonly needed to cover superficial injuries such as abrasions, cuts, bites, stings, reactions, or burns. The wound is best cleansed or soaked and an appropriate ointment (burn cream, antibiotic ointment, steroid cream, etc.) is applied to the affected area before applying a bandage. Eye patches are available in most pharmacies and are best for the eyes due to their nonabrasive material.

Steri-strips or bandage sutures are excellent to close small lacerations. They work best on dry skin and are especially effective in holding a wound closed if used with a liquid adhesive such as tincture of benzoin. It is important to inspect the laceration before closing it to be sure there are no foreign bodies in the tissues. Even jagged or uneven lacerations can be temporarily closed with steri-strips.

There are a variety of tapes that are applicable for wound care. Patients may have allergies to any of them. Allergies may be due to the material of the tape or the glue it possesses. Some of the stronger tapes are the silk and cloth tapes. Silk tape holds better with more effective glue. Paper tape is not as strong but has the lowest incidence of allergies reported. It is also the easiest to tear, although the silk and cloth tapes will tear in a straight line, even along their length. Paper tape must be cut with scissors if a straight edge is needed. Foam-backed tape will stretch and maintain some pressure on a wound. It is easy to tear and again must be cut with scissors if a straight edge is desired. Foam, silk, and cloth tapes will keep a wound somewhat drier and adhere better than paper tape in a wet environment.

Some of the tools that may be useful in times of emergency are a pair of scissors, forceps, clamps, hemostats, knife, scalpel, thermometer, pocket mask, tweezers, magnifying glass, bulb syringe, needle syringe, bowl or basin, cup, and matches. Scissors are needed to cut clothing or exposure suits away from a wounded area. This is the preferred method to clear the victim's body of clothing or dive wear. The cloth may be needed for other purposes so it is not discarded. Cutting string or rope may also be accomplished with heavy-duty shears. Clamps, hemostats, and forceps may be used to hold cloth or string together. They are extremely useful for clamping off bleeding vessels in deep wounds. They can be precisely placed on the artery or vein with accuracy. These useful tools can be used to grasp and peel containers or other objects. Foreign bodies in wounds can be debrided if need be. Tourniquets, if absolutely needed, can be made with a piece of cloth or rope and a snap that is rotated until the bleeding slows or stops.

Tweezers are useful for a variety of purposes. Wounds can be inspected and debrided with fine and blunt tweezers. Packing a wound with gauze is facilitated with tweezers. Handling injury site waste is preferred with an instrument and gloves. Removing wood, glass, or metal splinters is made much easier with a fine pair of tweezers. The magnifying glass can be used to better identify foreign bodies in a wound. It is very helpful when removing splinters, thorns, or stingers, and can assist in identifying small organisms or inspecting injuries. A bulb syringe can be used for irrigating the eyes if exposed to a toxic substance. It can also be used for irrigating a wound. Lavaging someone in hyperthermia with cold water can be done with a bulb syringe. Aspirating blood or fluid from a wound can be performed as well.

Checking a victim's vital signs may be made more precise with the proper tools. The thermometer is essential if fever, hyperthermia (overheating), or hypothermia (too cool) is suspected. A portable blood pressure monitor cuff may be needed for a variety of injuries causing internal and external bleeding. Blood pressure monitoring may be useful for victims of poisoning and venoms that cause anaphylactic shock, hypothermia and hyperthermia, lung expansion injuries, chest and abdominal injuries, heart attacks, and many other conditions. A stethoscope will make checking the heart rate and rhythm easier and listening to the lungs much more accurate.

Latex gloves and masks provide protection to the caregiver during treatment of any wound or when exposed to any body fluid. There are non-latex gloves that are now recommended because of the recently recognized increased incidence of latex allergies. Masks that have clear plastic eye protection are preferred. An alternative may be to use goggles with a mask that has no eye shield. Plastic bags and a biohazard label are advised for any and all waste generated by an emergency.

Suture material is quite useful if dealing with injuries, but its use should be limited to experienced medical personnel. There are different types of suture materials intended for different applications. There are monofilament fibers that have less area for bacteria to cause infection, or braided fibers that have better friction to hold strong knots. There are absorbable materials that are used internally that over several weeks dissolve, and non-absorbable materials such as nylon, silk, and wire. Suture materials are available without a needle for tying things or they are available on straight and curved needles for suturing. The particular tissue being sutured and the purpose of the stitch will dictate what type of stitch one is to use. The different types of stitches are the simple loop, mattress stitch, the horizontal mattress stitch, the figure eight, the continuous versus the interrupted, the inverted versus the conventional, etc. The different knots that can be used will depend on their application. Sutures are useful to stop bleeding, close or approximate gaping wounds, and support or approximate mutilated tissue. If a trained individual were present, suture would be a great adjunct to the medical kit.

TABLE 1
FIRST AID KIT

CREAMS and OINTMENTS
- a. Sun Screen
- b. Burn Cream
- c. Antibiotic Cream
- d. Anesthetic Cream
- e. Moisturizer
- f. Lip Balm*
- g. Petroleum Ointment*

MEDICATIONS
- a. Anti-metics (Anti-nausea)
- b. Analgesics (Pain Medication)
- c. Ethyl Alcohol
- d. Hydrogen Peroxide
- e. Ammonia
- f. Betadine™ Solution
- g. Benadryl™
- h. Oxygen Tank**
- i. Saline Eyewash
- j. Local Anesthetic* **
- k. Epinephrine* **
- l. Antibiotics* **
- m. Anti-venom **
- n. Intravenous Saline **
- o. Ice*

BANDAGES and BRACES
- a. Ace Wraps™
- b. Ankle Brace
- c. Splint
- d. Knee Brace
- e. Gauze (folded and rolled)
- f. Bandages (large and small)
- g. Tape
- h. Tincture of Benzoin
- i. Tourniquet
- j. Cotton Swabs
- k. Eye Pads
- l. Steri-Strips Bandage Sutures

INSTRUMENTS and TOOLS
- a. Scissors
- b. Forceps
- c. Hemostats
- d. Snaps
- e. Knife
- f. Scalpel* **
- g. Thermometer
- h. Pocket Mask
- i. Tweezers
- j. Magnifying Glass*
- k. Bulb Syringe
- l. Syringe* **
- m. Needles* **
- n. Graduated Cup*
- o. Bowl*
- p. Basin*
- q. Suture* **
- r. String
- s. Blood Pressure Monitor*
- t. Stethoscope*

PROTECTIVE ACCESSORIES
- a. Mask
- b. Glove (Non-latex Recommended)
- c. Eye Protection (Goggles)
- d. Plastic Bag (large)
- e. Biohazard Label*
- f. Towel
- g. Blanket
- h. Treatment Manual/Slates

COMMUNICATION EQUIPMENT
- a. Emergency Action Plan Sheet
- b. Ship to Shore Radio
- c. Portable Phone
- d. Emergency Procedures Checklist

*Recommended but not essential
**Only to be used by trained individuals

Floats/Buoys

Having several types of buoys and floats for different purposes is vital to safe boating and diving. It is mandatory by law in the U.S. and most other countries that there be at least one life vest on a boat for every passenger. The PFDs (Personal Flotation Device) must have the seal of approval from the U.S. Coast Guard to be valid in the U.S. The Code of Federal Regulations requires that the PFDs meet their requirements which includes having a minimum surface area of reflective material on the front (near the shoulders) and on the back and an approved waterproof light. The light may be chemical or battery. The chemical lights must be within three years of manufacture and the batteries for the battery-powered lights must be dated. The PFDs must have the name of the vessel printed or stamped on them. This will identify the vessel that the victims originated from. The PFDs must be stored on the upper decks in a location accessible to all passengers and not stacked more than 4 feet high. It is also required that the life vests aboard must fit the passengers present. It is therefore wise to have a variety of sizes and several vests in each size. At least 10% of the PFDs must be for children and must be stored separately from the adult vests to avoid confusion. It is my preference to also fasten a whistle to each life vest. The reader is encouraged to review the Code of Federal Regulations to be sure their PFDs comply with the requirements.

A lifeboat (or several lifeboats) may also be required depending on the size of the vessel and the number of passengers. Each lifeboat must have four paddles or oars (with the name of the vessel written on them), a sea anchor, a knife, and the name of the vessel written in letters at least two inches (5.1 centimeters) in height, and a waterproof light. The specifications of the lifeboats may be found in the Code of Federal Regulations.

A current line tied to a float preferably equipped with a small dive flag is an asset to every boat dive and some shore dives.

In a current, the diver can grasp the line (preferably knotted) to remain away from the back of the boat without drifting away or having to swim to stay in proximity of the boat. This allows divers to avoid injury as equipment is being handed in or out of the boat and while divers are entering or exiting the water. Current lines are also necessary during wavy conditions. It is unsafe to try to hold on to a swim platform or the back of a boat that is rocking. Severe head, neck, and/or extremity injuries could occur from a swim platform, a ladder, the hull of the boat, or a propeller blade coming down on a diver in high waves. During shore dives this flagged float can be used to warn boat traffic of dive operations close to shore and may be used by the divers to identify the exit site. This line may also be used to pull a diver into shore.

The Code of Federal Regulations requires a vessel to possess a throwable flotation ring at least 24 inches in diameter attached to a line at least 60 feet long. If the vessel is greater than 65 feet, three life rings are required. If the vessel is on inland waters the ring must be white, and if on coastal waters the ring must be orange. A life ring is also highly recommended for every shore dive. This may be used as the current line while shore diving. The line attached to the ring is preferably a buoyant rope (such as polypropylene) so that it will be more accessible to the divers if the buoy is thrown past them. When throwing the buoy to a diver or swimmer in trouble, try to throw the buoy or ring well past them and slightly toward the windward side, then pull it to the individual so they may be able to grasp the line or the ring. This will also ensure you do not under-throw the ring or strike the diver's or swimmer's head or face with the ring. The tired or incapacitated diver is not to pull himself or herself in; the rescuer should pull the diver in at a moderate rate so as not to pull the rope or ring out of the hands of a diver whose problem may not be readily apparent to the rescuer. If the diver does not grasp the line or is unable to get to the line, the rescuer is to immediately go in after them without delay. Repeated attempts at throwing a life ring at a disabled diver or swimmer may be futile and a waste of valuable time. The throwable flotation ring must to be kept on deck in a secure but accessible location.

It is recommended to have a marker buoy at hand on all dive boats. A weight with a line connected to a float or buoy can be kept in a bucket or rolled in some fashion. These units can be made or bought already assembled and kept on deck ready to be thrown in if something drops in and sinks. These handy buoys are perfect for marking a wreck site, a passage through a breakwater or reef, or just marking the spot where equipment or a diver has been lost. At night or late afternoon near sunset one can connect a lamp to the buoy or float (it could even be a dive flashlight or strobe light) to aid in identification of the location of the buoy in the dark.

The sausage buoy is an indispensable tool and doesn't inconvenience the diver in any way, and may be the only way in rough water or high seas that the diver may be spotted from the bridge of a boat or from shore. This visual distress tool is considered mandatory on all open-water dives. One could also use the sausage buoy for additional buoyancy if needed.

TABLE 2
FLOATS/BUOYS

a.	Life Vests	e.	Raft/Life Boat
b.	Life Ring	f.	Marker Buoy
c.	Current Line	g.	Buoyant Straps & Small Floats
d.	Sausage Buoy	h.	Resealable Plastic Bags

Having small floats for accessories is also a good idea. Having keys on a float is a staple routine for boaters. Everyone on a boat may benefit from this maritime custom. The use of floatable straps for glasses or sunglasses is recommended for obvious reasons. Putting binoculars, cameras, or other items on lanyards with floats is a sound practice. There are moderately heavy plastic bags for clothing and other items. These bags can be folded or sealed in some manner that makes them waterproof and buoyant. Pagers, hand-held GPS units, hand-held ship to shore radios, wallets, cameras, snacks, and portable phones can be placed in Ziploc™ plastic bags and kept dry and buoyant by sealing in some air in the bag. The pagers, radios, GPS and phone can even be used without having to open the bags. In this manner they can even be kept and used while on a personal watercraft or life raft.

Vessel Electronics

Even if the intended dive site were very close, a dive-boat would be better protected having a minimum stock of electronics equipment and gauges. This includes a portable phone and ship to shore radio for communication. A hand-held, battery-powered radio may not have the range that an onboard radio with a tall antenna will have but can be used in case of power failure and may be taken on a raft in case of sinking of the vessel. A radio log is required to record any distress calls one hears or receives and must be kept for at least three years. Distress signals sent by radio also need to be logged in the radio log. Channels 12 and 16 are for emergency use only. The improper use or use of profanity on the radio carries a $5,000 maximum fine. Instruments intended for positioning and piloting the vessel include a depth sounder, GPS (Global Positioning System) or Loran, and radar. A spare hand-held GPS is recommended in case of a power failure or use on a raft. Equipment needed to monitor engine status includes a speedometer, engine temperature gauges, gas gauge, and oil pressure gauges. Fish-finders or 3-D bottom readers can come in handy when searching for wrecks or specific bottom topography.

It is my personal preference to also include an AM/FM radio that can give weather information and a CD player for entertainment. In vessels with a cabin, an operational carbon monoxide detector increases the safety of the cabin. A hailer or megaphone can come in handy at times; many models include foghorns and sirens as well. A horn (whistle) and bell are required on any vessel 12 feet (3.7 meters) or greater for communicating with other vessels (or shore) at night or during limited visibility, while under way or while at anchor. The vessel needs to be equipped with the proper running lights and an anchor light. A bright spotlight for illumination, searches, and visualization is useful. As basic as it may seem, several good flashlights and battery-powered lamps are a necessity on a boat. An electric air pump and a foot pump in case there is no power for inflating a raft or tube may be needed.

TABLE 3
VESSEL ELECTRONICS

a. Ship to Shore Radio	b. Portable Phone
c. Hailer	d. Horn
e. GPS	f. Radar
g. Speedometer	h. Engine Temp Gauge
i. Oil Pressure Gauge	j. Gas Gauge
k. Depth Sounder	l. Fish Finder/Bottom Reader
m. AM/FM Radio	n. CD/Tape Player
o. Spot Light	p. Flash Lights
q. Battery Powered Lamps	r. Running/Anchor Lights

Vessel Equipment

A well-prepared vessel will need several items in addition to the electronics to optimize safety for its passengers and to comply with the law. Fenders of the proper size for the vessel are essential for pulling up to a wall or piling. Occasionally fenders may be needed to raft off another vessel. In open water it is best to transfer passengers or equipment as may be needed when rafting off another vessel, but quickly untie and allow the boats to float away from each other when diving. Wave conditions may change and boat damage may ensue from rafted vessels. Even during flat and calm conditions vessel damage may occur from the waves of distant bypassing boats.

A flare gun with fresh flares is also necessary. Keep the expired flares for spares rather than discarding them. Depending on the size of the boat, a number of fire extinguishers (checked monthly and inspected annually) are required as well as an extinguishing system in the engine compartment (Halon extinguishing systems have been phased out as of the year 2000). It is wise to have an emergency leak repair kit on any vessel. This may be comprised of a set of various sized wooden or rubber corks, a large tube of underwater compound, duct tape, rags, a waterproof tarp, epoxy, and possibly a fiberglass repair kit.

A vessel must display several items. It is necessary by law to have a sign prohibiting oil and gas discharge near the engine compartment as well as a sign in a visible location on the vessel prohibiting garbage dumping over-board. If the vessel is documented, the documentation papers (or copies) need to be onboard. The captain must have his or her captain's license available. A permit from the Department of Conservation allowing the vessel to carry charters should also be available if appropriate. The state registration sticker and the ship's registration numbers are to be displayed on both sides of the bow at least four inches in height. Keeping a copy of the vessel's insurance policy onboard may be considered.

Several appropriately sized ropes will be needed. Rope is made up of several different types of material. They are all fabricated in a similar fashion. The basic element is the material fiber that is woven into yarn which is then woven into strands that in turn are woven into rope. The materials for making rope are either natural (hemp, manila, cotton, and sisal) or synthetic materials that for the most part have replaced natural fibers. The synthetic fibers are polypropylene (olefin), polyester, polyamide (nylon), polyethylene, and aramid (kevlar). The polypropylene and polyethylene ropes float whereas all the others do not. Materials that float are excellent for rescue and for buoys, but should not be used for anchorage in ports to avoid entanglements with boat propellers. Nylon ropes are stronger and in general have better stretching properties than hemp. Nylon also resists rot better and lasts several years longer than hemp ropes. Nylon does have the disadvantage of degrading in sunlight over time.

There are two main types of rope and cable construction: the twisted rope type and the braided rope type with an external braided covering (sheath) and an inner or middle core that is also braided. The strength of the braided type of rope lies solely with the core. The braided rope can possess major frays in the inner core that may be hidden by the outer sheath. Some braided rope may hide a core that is made of a cheaper and less desirable material; this is known as "cheating" in the rope and boating industry. Braided rope is much softer and if pre-stretched does not expand any further. The twisted rope is less flexible and more applicable for heavy work and grips a knot much better than braided line.

Elasticity is just as important as the strength of the rope. An elastic material can absorb shock loads much better than a stiff, stronger rope. Polypropylene and nylon have the best elasticity of all ropes. Elasticity may pose certain risks. A nylon rope that parts (breaks) if stretched more than 40% of its length can snap back with the velocity of a .45 caliber bullet and cause significant injury. Standing aside instead of inline with the rope is recommended. Doubling the diameter of a rope will quadruple its strength. Always rinse and dry a rope before storing to prevent rot and mildew.

All divers and boaters should know a few basic knots to accomplish a variety of functions. Practice and experience in rope handling will be needed to maintain confidence and proficiency.

An anchor is considered basic boat equipment and the type of anchor should be appropriate for the local bottom composition of the body of water to be navigated. The size of the anchor should be appropriate for the size and weight of the vessel. A second anchor may be helpful to stabilize the vessel in waves or to add purchase to the vessel's primary anchor in wind or currents. A ladder at the stern to climb onto larger dive boats with or without a swim platform from the water must be available for divers. The ladder with the center pole design does have the advantage of allowing the diver to step up and climb the steps with fins donned.

TABLE 4
VESSEL EQUIPMENT

a. Fenders
b. Flair Gun
c. Fire Extinguishers
d. Engine Room Extinguisher
e. Emergency Leak Repair Kit
f. Notices Against Littering
g. Vessel Papers (documentation and registration papers)
h. Insurance Policy
i. Captain's License
j. Lines/Ropes
k. Anchors
l. Ladder

Essential Diving Gear

Diving requires a minimum stock of equipment that is needed for safety of the diver. This gear may be divided into categories of equipment for breathing, buoyancy control, propulsion, communication, and safety. Essentials needed for breathing include an air tank, snorkel, regulator, and octopus. Buoyancy control gear includes a buoyancy compensation device, belt, and weights. Fins are essential for propulsion while diving. Minimum communication tools for the surface and while submerged include the mask, tank banger, whistle, and the slate. Necessary safety equipment includes the depth gauge, tank pressure gauge, compass, watch, sausage buoy, and knife/tool. Equipment that is felt to be highly recommended to have while diving but not pertinent for every dive would include a self-contained ascent bottle, lamp, dive computer, gloves, boots, air horn, dive skin or wet suit, dive table/wheel, water temperature gauge, and electronic underwater communicators. A reel may be needed in case a diver is lost and a search is begun.

Going diving with fewer than the complete list of essential equipment will leave the diver less than prepared for the majority of adverse circumstances commonly encountered while scuba diving. Each of the listed items performs a vital function either during routine diving or during an emergency while in the water.

There are a few general recommendations that can be made concerning the care of diving equipment. It is not uncommon for a diver to leave a dive site missing a piece of equipment or with an extra glove or boot that belongs to another diver. For this reason it is recommended you label all of your gear with a permanent marker or label. Writing the owner's initials or name on every item will simplify the identification of a diver's equipment. A careful inventory of one's gear should be done before leaving for a dive and before anyone leaves the dive site.

TABLE 5
ESSENTIAL DIVE EQUIPMENT

Recommended but not essential for every dive

a. Mask	b. Fins	c. Snorkel
d. BCD	e. Weights	f. Air Tank
g. Knife/Tool	h. Whistle	i. Sausage Buoy
j. Slate/Pencil	k. Depth Gauge	l. Tank Pressure Gauge
m. Compass	n. Regulator/Octopus	o. Watch
p. Tank Banger	q. Lamp	r. Dive Computer*
s. Self-contained Ascent Bottle*	t. Gloves*	u. Boots*
v. Air horn*	w. Skin or Wetsuit*	x. Dive Table/Wheel*
y. Electronic Communicators*	z. Water Thermometer*	aa. Reel*

If all dive gear is periodically inspected and maintained, it will deliver safe and consistent function. Constant attention to cleanliness helps to keep one's gear smelling fresh, prolongs gear life, and prevents health risks. Many products are available for washing wet suits and gear. It matters less which product is used rather than that all gear is routinely washed and thoroughly dried.

The diver should make a conscious effort to obtain equipment that is brightly colored to make the diver as visible as possible. As recreational divers we need to be as conspicuous as we can. A Divemaster will have an easier time keeping track of a group, and a buddy will be able to be visualized at a greater distance. If wearing black or dark colors and lost or trapped, the "stealth look" may hinder a search. If gear is dropped overboard, bright- or neon-colored equipment will be easier to see from a distance, hence increasing the likelihood of being found.

Boating and Diving Accessories

Boating Accessories

There is an assortment of items and tools that is needed for a variety of circumstances that may be encountered during a boating excursion or diving trip. The most commonly needed tools to fix or adjust diving equipment or perform boat repairs include several pliers, channel locks, bolt and pipe wrenches (large and small), Allen wrenches, and an assortment of screwdrivers. A strong pair of scissors and a Swiss army knife are used more often than one may imagine. Spare hose clamps may also come in handy as would spare hoses for the engine compartment. A few spare quarts of motor oil onboard during an excursion is always a good idea as is Super glue™, and electrical and duct tape.

A set of local maps and navigational charts including navigational tools (dividers, parallel ruler, and compass) are fundamental for any excursion. Every vessel should also carry an updated copy of the Coast Pilot and the Light list in addition to the latest issue (weekly) of the Local Notice to Mariners. These issues will keep the boat operator updated concerning any changes or hazards in the navigable channels and waterways.

Sunglasses will help protect the eyes from UV rays and add to the comfort level in bright sunshine. Polarized lenses may also help filter out glare and aid in detecting debris, buoys, lines, or a diver on the surface or just under the surface of the water. Binoculars will help provide improved visibility for the Divemaster on board during a search for buoys, mooring lines, bubbles, divers, other boats, or shoreline. Infrared and "night vision" binoculars are useful for finding divers or objects at night.

Diving Accessories

Small metal picks can be used to remove O-rings and other small items during repair. Neoprene glue for repairing wet suits and silicone lubricant for keeping rubber seals on lights, cameras, and other containers waterproof should be available. If one is diving in remote areas where quality control is not practiced or is questionable, the use of carbon monoxide sensors is advised. There are several on the market and a supply to last the trip should be brought along.

A supply of zip-ties are needed for securing the regulator mouthpiece, octopus mouthpiece, BCD oral inflator, and fastening an assortment of tools, accessories, and slates to the hoses or D-rings. Adapters that attach to the BCD inflation hose for inflating inner tubes, floats, and rafts are handy tools to keep. You may want to bring an extra tank if inflating equipment is anticipated.

A dive flag is mandatory when divers are below. An international dive flag (blue and white flag also known as Code Flag A or Alpha) not less than one meter (about 3 feet) in height is the only federally approved flag (day shape) during dive operations, although many states will accept the conventional white diagonal stripe on red dive flag. The higher the flag is hung and the larger the flag, the better the visibility from a distance. Smaller flags on poles for inner tubes may be also considered and placed on the end of a current line or a line attached to a buddy team.

A five to seven foot long buddy line is good to have in cases of very poor visibility. Mask defogger should be brought on all dives. A dive table or dive wheel is needed on every dive trip. Lift bags of various sizes may also be required on some search and recovery dives. Lift bags with purge valves are recommended. Practice and training in their use is advocated to assure controlled ascents. Reels are an important piece of equipment especially for missing diver scenarios in poor visibility and search and recovery dives. Reels are also needed for wreck or cave and cavern diving. Metal detectors are useful on wreck or search and recovery dives.

Photographic equipment is a very applicable accessory to have on a dive trip. Since I do not advocate hunting or violating artifacts at a wreck site or any dive, a camera or video will capture the moment so one can share the experience with others without negatively impacting the dive site. A variety of equipment is available and is priced according to its quality and versatility. Adequate lighting is important and the clarity of the water will determine the depth of field one can obtain. Floating particles are notorious for reflecting the flash back to the camera and ruining one's pictures. Be careful not to get too close to some marine animals to photograph them. The flash may startle them and you may get more than just a picture. Be sure to have a lanyard or strap on the camera to prevent losing it. The Divemaster may consider taking along a camera or video or have a fellow diver film the dive and offer the tape to the divers. This is an easy way to add to the revenue without much effort and the divers usually cherish these tapes. Having a crew member do the filming allows the Divemaster to attend to shepherding the divers.

Another advancement in marine information is the availability of compact discs that contain programs indicating the type of flora and fauna that inhabit the oceans and seas at specified depths. These programs include photographs, scientific names (genus/species), physical descriptions, and other pertinent information. If a diver sees a fish and wants to identify it, they can input the physical characteristics and location into the laptop or PC and the program will locate a list of fish that fit the description. Books or slates for fish, creature, coral, and sponge identification are great substitutes to the digital programs. The photographs will assist the diver in making positive identification. I have found this practice very educational, entertaining, and an aid to more accurately logging the events and encounters of each dive.

Many establishments will require logbooks and most demand a certification card to take one diving. If the diver has a Divemaster card but is not in charge of the group, he or she may decide to use his or her non-professional certificate (i.e., Master scuba diver certificate) to limit legal entanglement if an injury were to occur to one of the divers during the dive. Insect repellent can aid in avoiding the annoyance and risk of disease transmitted by biting insects during pre-dive, surface interval, and post-dive periods. Additional items will obviously be added to the list depending on one's diving practices.

TABLE 6
DIVING AND BOATING ACCESSORIES

Boating
a. Pliers (several sizes)
b. Screwdrivers (all types and sizes)
c. Pipe Wrenches (all sizes)
d. Allen Wrenches
e. Channel Locks
f. Local Map and Nav. Charts
g. Motor Oil
h. Spare Engine Hose and Hose Clamps
i. Tape (duct tape and electrical)
j. Super Glue™
k. Sunglasses
l. Binoculars
m. Night Vision Binoculars
n. Camera

o. Insect Repellent
p. Knife
q. Scissors
r. Swiss Army Knife

Diving
a. Spare Tank (for inflating equipment)
b. Metal Picks
c. Mask Defogger
d. Carbon Monoxide Sensors
e. Dive Tables/Wheel
f. Neoprene Glue
g. Certification Card
h. Logbook

i. Lift Bag
j. Buddy Line
k. Dive Flags
l. Reel
m. Video Camera
n. Inflation Adapters (for tubes and rafts)

o. Silicone Lubricant
p. Fish Identification CD
q. Zip-ties

NOTES

CHAPTER TWO

Medical Examination

Management of any medical emergency requires three basic components: recognition and identification of the problem, a treatment plan, and the tools to carry out the treatment. A rescuer must rely on a victim's symptoms (what the victim is experiencing) and signs (what the rescuer observes on examination) in order to make a diagnosis. Knowledge of what is normal is required to determine if something is abnormal. The combination of the history (events leading up to the condition) and the physical findings will lead the rescuer to narrow down the possibilities of what is the cause of the victim's condition. Many times the most effective therapy is not treating the symptom, but rather correcting the cause.

If an injured diver or passenger is a member of the Divers Alert Network (DAN), the DAN number may be contacted along with the local EMS if circumstances indicate the need for further or more advanced medical care. Remember that the emergency contact person that the injured diver has listed for himself or herself is also to be notified of the emergency.

Physical Examination

Vital Signs
The vital signs are the four parameters that can be measured that are most important to survival of a person. These four parameters are respiration, heart rate, blood pressure, and temperature. Major deviations from normal of any of these four parameters would be considered life threatening. CPR (cardiopulmonary resuscitation) is devised to artificially attempt to correct all but the person's temperature. There is a range that is considered normal of these parameters. Knowing the ranges of normal would be important to identify which individual may require treatment or CPR.

The normal ranges of the vital signs are as follows:
- **Respirations** — 12 to 20 breathes per minute
- **Heart rate** — 60 to 100 beats per minute
- **Blood pressure** —100 to 140 mm of Hg (mercury) systolic
   — 60 to 90 mm of Hg (mercury) diastolic
- **Temperature** — 97° to 100° F (about 36° to 38° C)

It is important to understand that although the above ranges are what the "average" person may consider normal at rest, there are frequent circumstances that one may encounter that deviate beyond the above ranges and still be normal for that particular individual. A common example is that of a highly athletic individual who may consistently run heart rates in the forties and be considered normal. Another example is that temperature recordings will deviate depending on how the person's temperature is taken. For instance, axillary temperatures (taken in the underarm) are usually one to two degrees cooler than oral temperature, which are one to two degrees cooler than rectal temperatures in the same individual.

•Respiration

Respiratory rates are routinely measured by observing the person as they inhale and exhale. If a victim is breathing and motion of the chest is minimal and difficult to count, the rescuer may place a small mirror or glass in front of the victim's nose and mouth to check for fogging of the mirror during exhaling. The rescuer may also listen to the chest with their ear or stethoscope to check for ventilation. Respiratory rates can be obtained by counting the number of breaths for fifteen seconds and multiply by four, or count for thirty seconds and multiply by two, or just count for one full minute.

Adequate breathing or ventilation is determined by moving an adequate volume of air into and out of the lungs every minute. Therefore, it is not just the number of breaths per minute that determine whether there is adequate ventilation, but also the volume of air moved with each breathe. If a victim appears to be moving minimal volumes of air with each breath, they may require rescue breathing even if the number of breaths per minute is within a normal range.

A victim who is breathing very rapidly is at risk of respiratory fatigue and may decompensate and require rescue breathing. They need to be monitored very closely. The rapid respiratory rate may be due to air hunger from a number of causes that may be affecting their ability to exchange gases within the lung. A collapsed lung, fluid in the lungs, a pulmonary embolus, toxicity from contaminated air, and many other causes could be the source of the problem. The rescuer must attempt to identify the cause from the circumstances surrounding the victim's injury. The likely cause should then be addressed in the most appropriate manner possible in the field until medical personnel arrive.

•Heart Rate and Blood Pressure

Heart rate and blood pressure are considered together because they are so dependent upon each other. The majority of divers do not have blood pressure monitoring equipment and therefore an estimate of blood pressure is as close as one can get in the field under these circumstances. Blood pressure monitors are commercially available for use in the field.

Both the heart rate and an estimate of blood pressure are usually obtained from monitoring the pulse of a victim. Pulses are felt where major arteries are close to the surface of the skin (See Figure 1 for location of pulses). The most commonly used pulses are the carotid pulse located on either side of the trachea, the radial pulse located on the inside of the wrist on the side of the thumb, the femoral pulse at the groin, and the pedal pulse on the top of the foot.

When attempting to feel the pulse, the rescuer should apply light pressure with the index and middle fingers only. Too much pressure may occlude the artery and obliterate the pulse. The index and middle fingers have the highest concentration of sensory organs and have a much better sense of touch than the other fingers. There is slight variability in all people and the pulse may be in a slightly different location from one individual to another. The rescuer should move the fingers lightly over the area of the pulse until the best location for the pulse is found.

Several parameters of the pulse rate can be obtained. The rate, the rhythm, and the strength of the pulse may give the rescuer information about the victim. The rate can be obtained by counting the pulses for fifteen seconds and multiplying by four, counting for thirty seconds and multiplying by two, or counting for one complete minute. The pulse rhythm should be regular. That is to say, the time interval between beats should be the same between all beats. An irregular rhythm could be a sign of heart disease, lack of oxygen, toxicity, or many other problems.

The strength of the pulse may give the rescuer an indication of the blood pressure and other important information. A strong pulse is indicative of good blood flow and pressure. A bounding pulse may indicate that the heart is strong but may be an early sign of blood loss or other causes of shock. A weak pulse may indicate late signs of shock due to a number of causes. A rescuer may elect to compare pulses at different sites. An injured extremity with swelling may have a diminished pulse due to compression of the artery by the swelling process or bleeding within that extremity, and may not reflect an accurate assessment of the victim's pulse or blood pressure.

• **Temperature**

Accurate temperature measurement of a victim can be obtained only with a thermometer. Touching the victim's forehead or neck is very unreliable. Even touching the victim's underarm or placing ones finger in the victim's mouth is not a reliable manner to assess temperature. There are many types of thermometers available that can easily obtain a victim's temperature. Temperature measurements can be obtained from the skin, tympanic, axillary, oral, and rectal readings. There are a multitude of problems and conditions that can alter all other temperature measurements other than rectal temperature recordings. The most important information for divers is their core temperature and the most accurate recording of core temperature is by rectal readings.

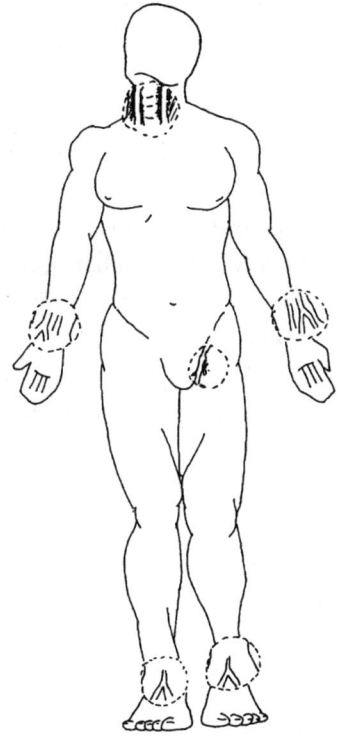

Figure 1 Location of Pulses.

Musculoskeletal System

Examination of the musculoskeletal system should follow an orderly pattern whether starting from the head down or from the feet upward. In the unconscious victim, this is more important than in an alert individual who can voice his or her complaints of pain, discomfort, or numbness. Attention may first be focused on areas where there is an obvious problem or complaint by the victim, but after that area has been evaluated the rescuer should then survey the rest of the anatomy for problems in an orderly fashion.

Exposure of the injured area should be done with gentleness and care. Minimizing movement of the injured region is important for the victim's comfort as well as preventing further injury. Cutting away the clothing or exposure suit is recommended to limit movement of the injured area. Complaints of pain or tenderness are the most reliable signs of an injury unless the neurological system has been affected.

•Extremities

Deformity of an extremity is an obvious sign of a fracture. Severe deformities may compromise blood circulation to the distal aspect of a limb and should be reduced to the most anatomical position possible. Minor deformities should be immobilized as they are. Swelling within a very short time period from the injury may be a sign of internal bleeding. Asymmetry with the other limb suggests a fracture although many individuals may have asymmetrical limbs. Abnormal position of the limb may indicate a fracture or torn ligaments at the joint where the abnormality is located. Shortening of a limb would suggest an impacted fracture until proven otherwise.

Massive hemorrhage into an extremity may cause a "compartment syndrome" and could compromise circulation to the distal aspect of the limb. Frequent checks of the distal pulses are recommended as well as expedient transfer to a medical facility.

Elevation of the limb may help reduce swelling and improve circulation. Discoloration may be a sign of several ominous complications. Ecchymosis (black and blue discoloration) is a sign of internal bleeding. This may occur early if the bleeding is just under the skin or may appear later if bleeding is deep and the blood slowly works its way to the surface. Cyanosis (bluish discoloration) of areas distal to the injury is a sign of lack of oxygenated blood in the extremity and is a true emergency. Blanching (pale discoloration) of the area distal to an injury reflects lack of circulation to that part of the extremity and is also a true emergency. Both of these signs of reduced or lack of circulation to the extremity may lead to loss of that limb if not treated immediately. Circulation to an extremity may be assessed by pressing on the fingernail or toenail and looking for return of pinkish color after releasing the pressure. If the nail bed does not have capillary refill of blood within one to two seconds the extremity is not adequately being perfused with blood flow.

- **Head**

Examination of the head includes looking for signs of bleeding from the surface and from any of the openings of the ears, nose, and mouth. Discoloration and tenderness are signs of injury. Swelling or indentations may be felt when lightly feeling the scalp. Inspection for facial trauma is done as well and is a common finding with head injuries. Evaluation of eye and jaw movement is done to rule out facial bone fractures. Asymmetry and tenderness of the cheekbones and the bridge of the nose may suggest other facial injuries or fractures. Bleeding into the conjunctiva (whites of the eye) or loss of vision from blood in the anterior chamber of the eye (hyphema) may be signs of ocular injury. Bleeding from the mouth may be due to tongue, gum, or tooth injury. Teeth may be knocked out and could result in aspiration of blood or the tooth causing severe coughing or respiratory difficulty. Bluish discoloration of the lips may be a sign of poor oxygenation due to lung or heart dysfunction.

Head injuries are frequently associated with spine and brain injuries and these need to be inspected and monitored. Specific head injuries are discussed below with their associated findings and management.

•Spine

If there is a potential spine injury, the victim should be placed on a straight and hard surface on their back. The head is placed and immobilized in a straight and neutral position. The rescuer may slide his or her hand beneath the victim, maintaining the spine as straight as possible to gently palpate (feel) each vertebral spinous process and check for tenderness. Swelling of an injured area is uncommon over the spine. The examiner may feel movement of a broken spinous process that is associated with pain. Spasms of the muscles on either side of the spine may be associated with spinal injuries or a soft tissue injury of the area. If a spine injury is suspected the individual should have a neurological exam performed and recorded.

Neurological Survey

Although it is important to obtain a thorough neurological survey, it is not necessary to obtain an extremely accurate neurological exam in the field. It is important, however, to be able to examine a victim and be able to assess the neurological status, and to determine the probable region of injury and take initial steps to prevent further damage. The neurological exam encompasses a variety of systems that may require other body systems to fully assess. For instance, it would be difficult to assess strength in an extremity with a broken bone. Assessing the neurological state of a victim will require taking the entire picture into consideration. Serial exams may be needed to document progression of injury in certain circumstances.

•Mental Status

Mental status evaluations of a victim determine whether the victim is awake or arousable, their level of orientation, and their ability to interact appropriately with their environment. Changes in mental status usually indicate either a structural or biochemical alteration within the brain. Bleeding within the brain, lack of blood flow to the brain, toxins, lack of oxygen, and, rarely, psychological causes may lead to mental status changes. Associated injuries, activities, and conditions will give leads as to the likely cause of the alteration.

If the victim is awake and able to verbalize, they may be asked their name, where they are, and what the date is. This will establish their orientation to person, place, and time. Memory may be evaluated by asking simple questions such as their birth date, family members' names, where they are staying, etc. Many victims may be uncooperative and recording their level of agitation, restlessness, or combativeness is also important. A short period of unconsciousness after a head injury would indicate a concussion and would be important information to disclose to medical personnel. Documentation of progression of lethargy or somnolence is also important for future care by medical personnel.

An unconscious victim may have reflex-type responses that give clues to the examiner about the location and type of injury. Rubbing the sternum with one's knuckles or pinching them on the arm are common methods of applying a noxious or painful stimulus to elicit a response. Recording their motor and verbal responses or lack thereof is very important. The Glasgow Coma Scale used in hospitals is based on patients' motor, verbal, and eye responses and is a good predictor of survivability of unresponsive victims. The victim is scored by the best response in each category and the scores are added together to give a final score.

TABLE 7
GLASGOW COMA SCALE

Eye Opening
- Spontaneous — 4
- To verbal stimulus — 3
- To pain — 2
- None — 1

Best Motor Response
- Obeys commands — 6
- Localizes to pain — 5
- Withdraws to pain — 4
- Abnormal flexion of arms — 3
- Abnormal Extension — 2
- None — 1

Verbal Response
- Oriented — 5
- Confused — 4
- Inappropriate words — 3
- Incomprehensible sounds — 2
- None — 1

The possible scores range from 3 to 15 and the lower the score, the worse the prognosis. A victim with a spinal cord injury may not be able to be assessed by this scale since motor function may be affected by the spinal trauma and would not reflect brain function.

• **Cranial Nerves**

There are twelve pairs of cranial nerves that are important because they originate directly within the brain, not from the spinal cord. All twelve pairs of these nerves pass through the skull to areas of the face and neck. Seven pairs of these cranial nerves serve functions in and around the eyes; therefore, the eye exam is quite important. The importance of abnormalities of these nerves is to identify problems within the skull and brain. The average diver need not memorize the names or functions of all the nerves but should be able to document abnormalities of the face and neck to pass the information on to future caretakers of the victim. Checking the pupils will establish if they are equal. Shining a light into the eyes may indicate whether they react to light by constricting and dilating once the light has been removed. Pupils that are unequal or completely dilated and non-reactive in an unresponsive victim are an ominous sign of severe brain dysfunction and impending death.

Table 8 is a review of the cranial nerves and their function.

TABLE 8

Cranial Nerve		Function
I.	Olfactory Nerve	Smell
II.	Optic Nerve	Sight
III.	Oculomotor Nerve	Moves eyes up, down, and inward, constricts pupil
IV.	Trochlear Nerve	Moves eyes down and inward
V.	Trigeminal Nerve	Sensation of cornea. Muscles of chewing
VI.	Abducens Nerve	Moves eyes outward
VII.	Facial Nerve	Closes eyelids. Movement of the facial muscles
VIII.	Vestibulocochlear Nerve	Hearing. Equilibrium and position of head
IX.	Glossopharyngeal Nerve	Sensation of tongue and throat, swallowing muscles
X.	Vagus Nerve	Controls heart rate. Sensation of ear and throat
XI.	Accessory Nerve	Neck muscles
XII.	Hypoglossal Nerve	Tongue muscles

•Motor

Evaluation of the motor system of the body may be made difficult because of associated injuries and the altered mental status of the victim. A motor deficit may occur from injuries of the brain, spine, peripheral nerve, or the muscle itself. There are several easy rules that may give the rescuer an idea where the injury may be that is affecting the motor system. There are many exceptions to these rules, but for the most part they can be used in a general way to understand why a victim may not be moving a part of his or her body. The circumstances surrounding the injury may add further clues to where the specific injury causing paralysis or weakness may be localized.

The brain is arranged in such a way that the body's motor function is controlled by the opposite side of the brain. A victim who has a motor deficit that affects the entire half of the body (face, arm, and leg) will most likely have an injury to the brain on the opposite side of the paralysis. Those individuals who have weakness or paralysis of the right side will likely have a speech problem as well because the speech centers are located on the left side of the brain in the majority of individuals. If the paralysis or weakness affects both sides of the body (either both legs or all four extremities) the injury is likely to be within the spinal cord. Sensation is usually affected along with the motor deficit, and mental status is normal in isolated spinal cord injuries. If the arms are affected the spinal injury is usually within the cervical spine (neck). If the victim is unable to breathe in addition to paralysis of all four extremities, it signifies a high cervical cord injury (above the fifth cervical vertebra). If the problem affects areas from the chest or belly down, the injury would usually be in the thoracic area of the spine (middle of the back). If the problem affects only the legs it is usually in the lumbar spine (low back). If a motor deficit is isolated to only one extremity the problem is likely to be within the nerve of that extremity (peripheral nerve injury).

The following crude method of measuring strength can be used in most circumstances. It is reproducible and understandable by most individuals.

- 0   No observable muscle contraction
- 1   Muscle contraction
- 2   Unable to overcome gravity
- 3   Able to overcome gravity
- 4   Slight weakness
- 5   Normal strength

•Sensation

There are numerous sensory organs that convey information to the brain within the skin, muscles, tendons, and internal organs. Pain is probably one of the most important sensations a person possesses as it allows the brain to immediately know where damage is occurring in the body. A rescuer can use information derived from the location of a victim's pain to identify injured areas. The rescuer is also interested in the ability of the victim to feel touch over the entirety of the body.

A rescuer may initially examine the victim's body by gently pressing and squeezing from the head down to determine if there is any tenderness over any parts of the body. Tenderness or pain will usually isolate areas of bruising, bleeding, or fracture. The rescuer should then use their finger or other soft object to ask if the victim has normal sensation over their body and document any areas lacking in sensation. If sensation is lacking, the rescuer can use the pattern of numbness to possibly identify the area of injury causing the sensory deficit. There may also be a motor deficit associated with the sensory deficit that would help identify the location of neurological system injury.

Sensory loss in the face is usually due to a brainstem insult or cranial nerve injury from a skull fracture. Numbness of the arms may indicate a cervical spine (neck) injury. If numbness is isolated to the arm, it may indicate a nerve root problem whereas if the rest of the body is also numb it would suggest a spinal cord injury. Sensory loss of the chest or belly may indicate a thoracic level spine injury (mid-back). Loss of sensation of the legs may only indicate a lumbar spine injury (low-back). Numbness of one extremity may be due to a nerve injury within the extremity itself.

•Cerebellar Function

The cerebellum is that part of the brain located in the back of the head. It is the coordination center for the body and controls the harmonious and smooth movements of all muscles to perform a task. Injury or damage to this part of the brain rarely causes numbness or significant weakness unless other areas of the brain are also affected, but will affect balance and coordination. In contrast to other functions of the brain, the cerebellum controls the muscles on the same side of the body. That is, the right cerebellum controls the right side of the body and the left cerebellum the coordination of the left side of the body.

A rescuer may ask the victim to alternate touching their own nose and then touching the rescuer's fingertip that is held about an arm's length away from the victim. This exam is referred to as the "finger-nose test" and is performed first using the victim's right then left arm. The test is abnormal if the victim consistently misses either the nose or the examiner's finger. Asking victims to stretch their arms out to their sides, close their eyes and touch their index fingers together in front of themselves performs another test. A normal individual may miss only once.

Other tests of cerebellar function are checking for rapid alternating movements such as rapidly tapping one's index finger to the victim's thumb, clapping, and tapping one's feet. Examination of how a victim walks may indicate a drunk-like gait, or inability to walk backward. Inability to tandem walk (walking on a straight line) is also a sign of potential cerebellar dysfunction.

CHAPTER THREE
Medical Management

Cardiopulmonary Resuscitation

It would be wise for any and all divers to know basic cardiopulmonary resuscitation (CPR). All certifying agencies do offer CPR and first aid courses. These are highly recommended.

When a victim is not breathing for a significant period of time, there is a high possibility the heart is not effectively beating either. A rescuer needs to check both the victim's respiration and pulse before beginning CPR. The rescuer must check to see if there is anything in the victim's mouth. The rescuer may check respirations by placing their ear near the mouth of the victim and listening for breath sounds, feeling for breath on the ear or cheek, and watching the chest wall for movement. An inadequate respiratory frequency (normal respiratory rate is 12 to 20 per minute) or moving an inadequate volume of air with each breath would be reason to initiate rescue breathing. The pulse can be checked in a variety of places on the body. The easiest are the carotid pulse on either side of the trachea (windpipe), the radial pulse just above the wrist on the side of the thumb, and the femoral pulse to either side of the groin region (See Figure 1 on page 31 for location of pulses). The pulse can tell the rescuer about the rate of the heart (normal being 60 to 100 beats per minute). A rapid pulse could indicate blood loss, anaphylactic shock, pain, and anxiety. A slow pulse could indicate a primary heart condition, or a toxin slowing the heart rate. A weak pulse could indicate significant blood loss or vascular relaxation such as in anaphylaxis. An absent pulse indicates cardiac arrest.

Before initiating CPR, call, shake, tap, pinch, or rub one's knuckle along the sternum of the victim and note their response. A rescuer should be able to observe breathing while checking for pulses. If the victim has inadequate or missing pulses or respirations, one should initiate CPR. The victim is placed on their back with arms at the side and legs straight and together. If there is a single rescuer, they are usually kneeling beside the victim's shoulder. A right-handed rescuer is usually on the victim's right side or vice versa for a left-handed rescuer (See Figure 2 for position to deliver rescue breaths in one-person CPR). Lifting the victim's jaw or slightly extending the neck if a spine injury is not a concern will help maintain the airway during rescue breathing. The nostrils are pinched with the rescuer's hand that is on the side toward the victim's head. The neck and back of the head are supported by the rescuer's hand that is on the side toward the victim's feet. The rescuer must place his or her mouth over the victim's mouth forming an airtight seal. The rescuer delivers two full breaths. The rescuer then moves slightly to a position beside the victim's chest (See Figure 3 for position to deliver chest compressions during one-person CPR). He or she then places the heal of the right hand (for a right-handed rescuer) on the sternum two finger-breadths above the lower edge of the sternum. With the heal of the left hand over the right hand, one pushes straight down about two inches (5 cm) to squeeze the blood in the heart out to circulate. The rescuer then quickly releases the pressure to allow the heart to fill again before the next compression. After fifteen compressions are delivered at a rate of about

MEDICAL MANAGEMENT

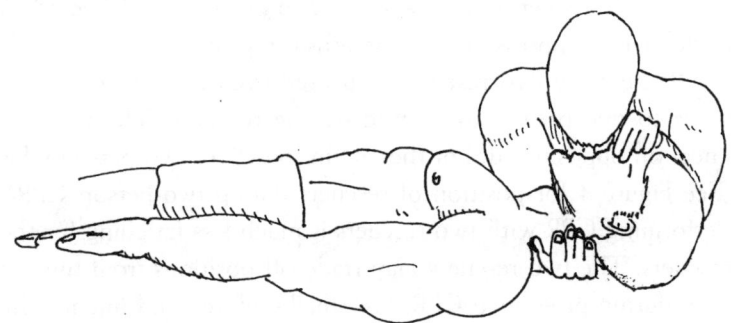

Figure 2 Position for delivering rescue breaths in one-person CPR.

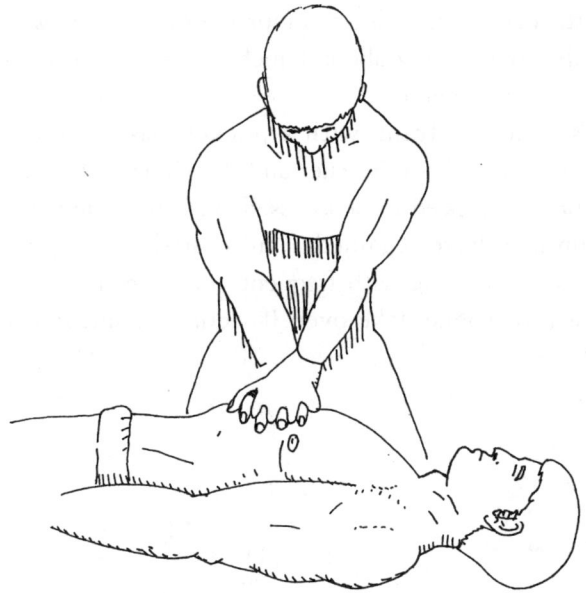

Figure 3 Position for delivering chest compressions during one-person CPR.

80 – 100 beats per minute, another two breaths are delivered. A cycle of 15 compressions to 2 breaths is repeated.

If there are two rescuers, repeated cycles of five compressions to one breath are shared by the rescuers. The rescuers kneel on opposite sides of the victim to deliver two-person CPR (See Figure 4 for position of rescuers during two-person CPR). Performing CPR with two rescuers is much less fatiguing for the rescuers. The two rescuers may trade off positions from time to time during prolonged CPR. For small children and infants, the rescuer covers the mouth and nose with their mouth in an airtight fashion and delivers small puffs of air at a rate of 20 to 30 breaths per minute. Chest compressions are done with the two thumbs compressing about 1 inch (2.5 cm) at a rate of 100 to 140 beats per minute.

Rescue breathing with a pocket mask maintains better hygiene for both the rescuer and the victim. The victim's pulse and breathing need to be assessed every five minutes or so. The victim may have regained a pulse or the ability to breathe. Careful monitoring with frequent vital signs is continued until medical personnel take over. If victims vomit, rescuers are to

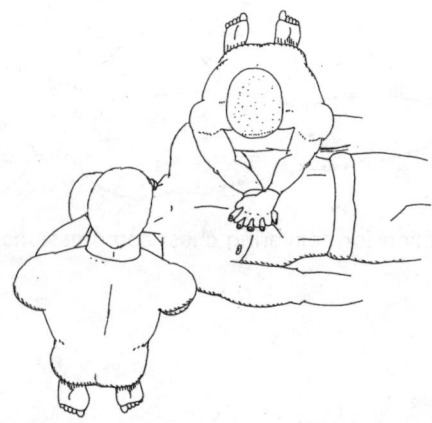

Figure 4 Position of rescuers during two-person CPR.

immediately turn them to the three-quarters prone position to prevent the vomit from entering their airway. Their mouths are cleaned as much as possible, and CPR is continued. (See Figure 14 on page 66 for Three-Quarter prone position.)

Airway Obstruction

If a victim is attempting to breath but is unable to move air in and out of the airway, or if an unconscious victim is unable to have rescue breathing delivered because of significant resistance, the airway may be obstructed by a foreign body. Other circumstances may be the cause, such as a tension pneumothorax (collapsed lung) or a hemothorax (bleeding into the chest cavity). The circumstances surrounding the injury may give leading clues as to the cause.

If an obstructed airway is suspected, the rescuer should sweep his or her finger deep in the back of the throat behind the tongue to attempt to dislodge the obstructing object. If the object is felt but unable to be removed or if nothing is felt, the rescuer should attempt a Heimlich maneuver (abdominal thrust). If the victim is conscious this is done by standing behind the victim, putting one's arms around the victim, and while holding one's hands together forcefully thrust inward and upward between the navel and the lower rib cage (See Figure 5 for Abdominal Thrust of Conscious Victim). This should be repeated several times until the

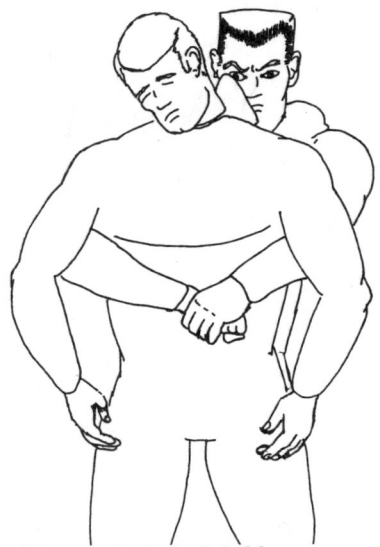

Figure 5 Heimlich Maneuver for Conscious Victim.

obstructing object is dislodged and the victim is able to breathe. Coughing by the victim is the first sign of an open airway.

If the victim is unconscious, the abdominal thrust is performed with the victim laying on their back and the rescuer sitting on their thighs facing the head of the victim (See Figure 6 for Abdominal Thrust of Unconscious Victim). The rescuer places one hand over the other just below the ribs and thrusts in and up. This is done as many times as may be necessary to dislodge the obstructing object. Once the object has been dislodged, quickly clear it from

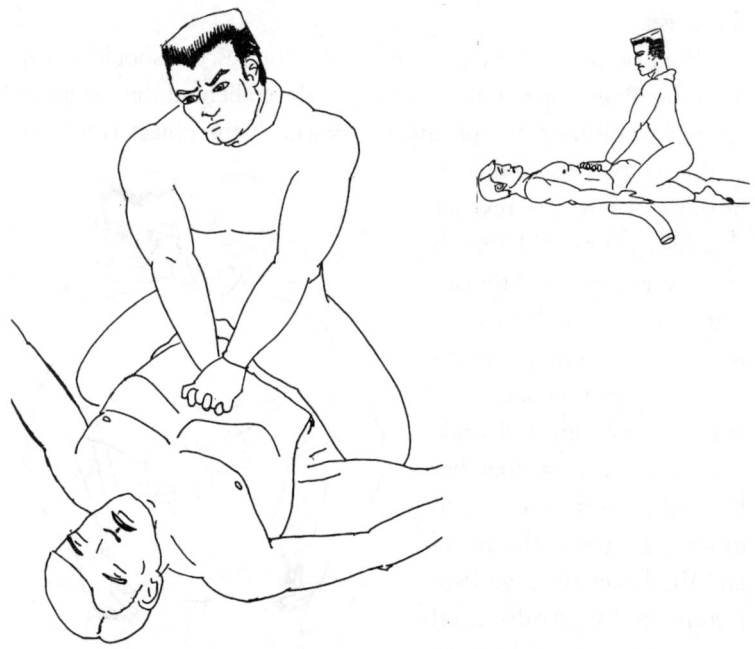

Figure 6 Abdominal Thrust for an Unconscious Victim.

the mouth of the victim before it lodges in the airway again. If the victim is either extremely obese or pregnant, the thrusts should be preformed as chest thrusts as if delivering CPR. Attempting rescue breathing after the above maneuvers may allow for adequate artificial ventilations by the rescuer.

Cricothyroidotomy

If all attempts at clearing the airway are unsuccessful, the rescuer should be familiar with performing an artificial airway, a cricothyroidotomy. This procedure is not recommended for victims while they are still conscious. Most victims would have lost consciousness by the time all the above maneuvers have been unsuccessfully attempted. The procedure is made easiest if a large bore hypodermic or spinal needle is available. If not, any thin, hard, hollow tool (i.e., broken radio antenna, straw, or pen barrel) will achieve the same result. Sterility is desired but in an emergency a life-saving artificial airway should be done despite sterility. A grateful survivor can always be treated later for an infection.

The victim is placed on their back with the head and neck slightly extended. The skin over the neck is then stretched tight over the thyroid cartilage (Adam's apple) (See Figure 7 for cricothyroidotomy procedure). Locate the V-shaped notch over the thyroid cartilage and slide down slightly to a space between the thyroid cartilage and the cricoid cartilage just below (See Figure 8 for Locating the Cricothyroid Membrane). This is the membrane that is to be penetrated by the needle. If a needle is not available the skin incision can be made with a pointed knife or scissors and the membrane punctured. Do not puncture the back wall of the trachea; penetrate only the sufficient depth to enter the airway. The hollow artificial airway may then be passed into the trachea (See Figure 9 for Placing Artificial Airway). Place antibiotic ointment around the artificial airway, cover with gauze, and secure with tape on either side of the neck.

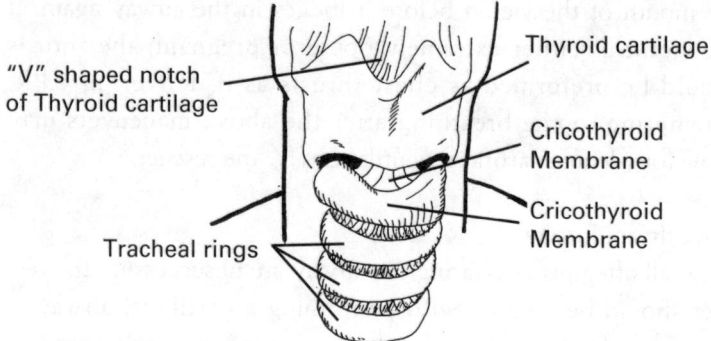

Figure 7 Front view of trachea and cricothyroid membrane.

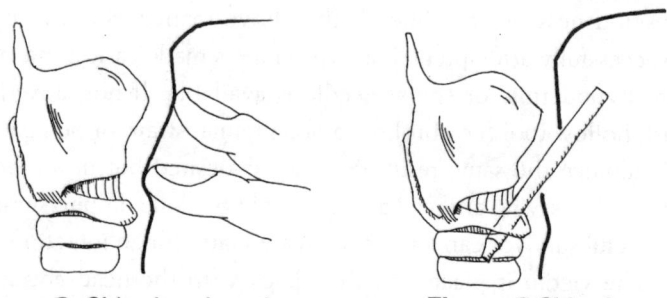

Figure 8 Side view: Locating cricothyroid membrane.

Figure 9 Side view: Inserting artificial airway.

If the victim begins to breathe on his or her own, supply oxygen to the end of the artificial airway. If the victim is not breathing, begin rescue breathing through the artificial airway. If rescue breathing is still not possible because the obstruction is lower than the artificial airway the rescuer may attempt to forcefully blow the obstruction down into one of the two main stem bronchi. The rescuer is to cover the artificial airway with their thumb and deliver a powerful breath by mouth-to-mouth breathing. If successful, this maneuver will at least allow for ventilation of one lung, which in most individuals should sustain life. If this is unsuccessful, it is doubtful the victim will survive.

Pneumothorax and Hemothorax

Pneumothorax is a collapse of the lung with free air within the chest cavity. Air trapped in the chest cavity under pressure can compress the lungs and prevent the lung from re-expanding (tension pneumothorax). A flap-like leak allows air to escape the lungs and fill the chest cavity but prevents its escape. The same can happen in precordial emphysema, where the heart is unable to fill with blood due to the pressure from air surrounding the heart. Blood circulation in the body will stop. Bleeding into the lungs and chest cavity can worsen this already bleak picture (hemothorax). Pneumothorax and hemothorax may be complications of crush or penetrating chest injuries as well as from decompression injuries.

Signs and symptoms can vary greatly depending on the size of the pneumothorax and the specifics of the affected diver or trauma victim. A diver with a collapsed lung most commonly has shortness of breath, rapid respirations or inability to inhale, chest pain, unresponsiveness, blue lips and nail beds (cyanosis), and coughing up blood (hemoptysis). Absent breath sounds on the affected side are the hallmark of a pneumothorax. Both the pneumothorax and the hemothorax will exhibit decreased breath sounds on the affected side of the chest associated with respiratory distress, difficulty in delivering rescue breathing, and a weak and rapid pulse. The difference on examination between a hemothorax and a pneumothorax is that with a pneumothorax the chest will sound hollow or tympanitic (like a drum) upon percussion (tapping the chest wall) whereas a hemothorax will sound dull or solid (full of fluid). Pneumothorax can be complicated by an air embolus. If the embolized air enters the arteries of the brain or the heart this could produce severe, sometimes fatal complications.

Unfortunately, few divers have the clinical experience to diagnose and treat this condition appropriately. The best treatment in the field by non-medical personnel is to administer 100% oxygen and treat the victim with CPR as required by the clinical presentation until emergency medical personnel arrive. If there is a very high degree of suspicion that a tension pneumothorax exists and the victim is rapidly deteriorating, the victim should have the chest cavity purged to reduce the pressure and allow for adequate inhalations and circulation.

Aspiration of the trapped air with a large bore syringe introduced into the chest cavity to the shallowest depth required to tap the air is the preferred method to relieve the pressure. The needle may be introduced into the chest cavity between the ribs at the level of the nipple, just lateral (to the side) of the pectoral muscle (See Figure 10 for location of needle insertion).

Sliding the needle just above the rib helps avoid puncturing the vein, artery, and nerve that run below each rib. The needle should not be moved side to side, only straight in and out, or lacerations of the lung can occur once it expands. The needle is advanced on an angle as the plunger of the syringe is aspirated (See Figure 11 for Insertion of Needle).

When the tip of the needle enters the air pocket, the plunger will suddenly pull out easily. If air is under pressure it will escape if the syringe is disconnected from the needle. This maneuver will not cure or eliminate the entire pneumothorax but will reduce the intra-thoracic pressure sufficiently to allow breathing and circulation until definitive medical management is given in a medical facility. If the air leak continues, the rescuer must continue to aspirate air or the tap may need to be repeated as circumstances dictate. It is also possible that the victim may have both lungs collapsed and require decompression of both sides of the

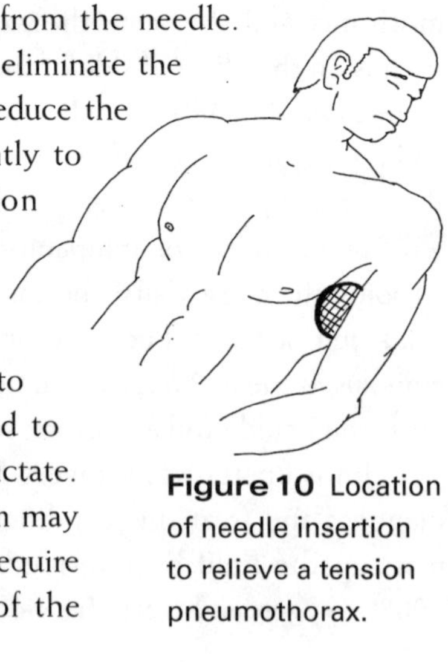

Figure 10 Location of needle insertion to relieve a tension pneumothorax.

chest cavity. When the needle is removed, it is to be pulled out quickly and pressure is placed over the puncture site for five to ten minutes to prevent bleeding.

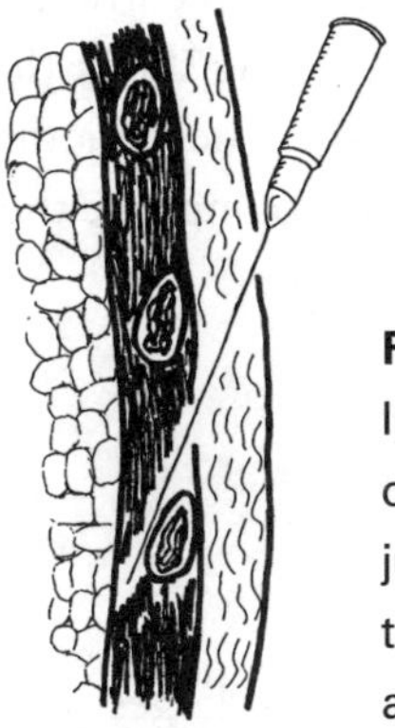

If a syringe is not available, a rescuer may need to puncture the chest cavity with a thin sharp instrument (i.e., Swiss army knife, fillet knife, pencil, antenna, etc.) to create the passage, then introduce a hollow instrument (i.e., straw, pen shaft, etc.) to relieve the pressure. Placing a flap valve on the hollow instrument will allow air to exit the chest cavity but prevent air from re-entering (See Figure 12 for Needle with Flap Valve). A flap valve can be made with a balloon that has a hole on the end or a latex glove finger with a small hole on the end. These may then be tied onto the end of the hollow instrument.

Figure 11 Insertion of needle just above the rib on an angle.

The alternate tools used for puncturing and tapping the trapped air must be sterilized as best as the circumstances will allow before their use. This can be done with alcohol, peroxide, or Betadine™ solution. These tools must be dried from these solutions before their use.

Drainage of the blood from the chest cavity requires a much larger opening than a needle and syringe will allow. An incision between the ribs and drainage of the blood is necessary. Rescue breathing will be required to reexpand the lung. Release of the blood from the chest cavity is almost always associated with

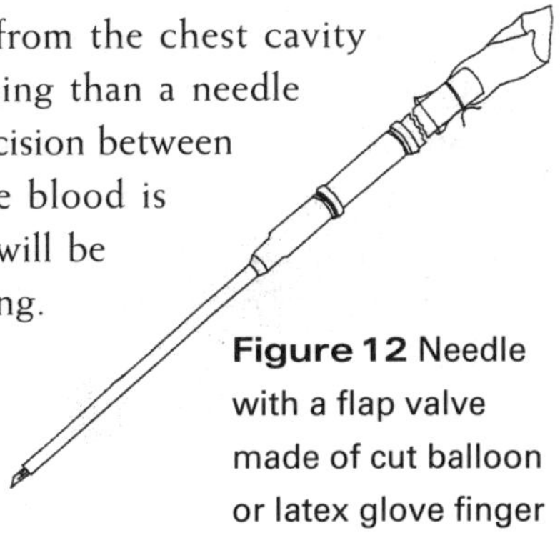

Figure 12 Needle with a flap valve made of cut balloon or latex glove finger tied to end of needle.

either continued or recurrent bleeding, and rapid blood loss may lead to hypovolemic shock (loss of blood pressure due to excessive blood loss). These victims require immediate surgery at a medical facility to improve their chances of survival.

Burns

Classification

The skin is the largest organ of the body. Amongst its many functions, the skin is the first line of defense against invasion by microorganisms and prevents loss of fluid by the body. Losses of these two functions are the leading causes of death from extensive burns. The depth and extent of surface area of the burned tissue is used to classify the severity of a burn. First-degree burns are superficial and involve only the epidermis. The skin may be reddened and painful but the skin is intact. The symptoms will resolve within 72 hours and the injury leaves no scar. The area may be treated with a cooling cream and covered with sterile gauze.

Second-degree burns involve the entire epidermis and partial thickness through the dermis (corium). Blistering is the hallmark sign of this type of burn but may not occur until later. Do not break the blister as this maintains sterility of the wound. Intense pain is the second sign of this type of injury. Cooling is very important to prevent deeper tissue damage. Fluid loss may be significant in victims with large surface areas involved. Scarring may be variable depending on the size and depth of the injury. Burn cream may be used or otherwise a dry sterile dressing is applied.

Third-degree burns are full-thickness injuries. In contrast to the other two categories where the burn will heal on its own, a third-degree burn will need a graft in most circumstances.

Scarring is extensive, and in sharp contrast to the more superficial burns, the area burned is painless and there is a lack of sensation. Pain is localized only to the edges of the burn. The charred skin should be left in place. After cooling the affected area a dry sterile dressing is applied. No creams or ointments are to be applied in the field. Avoid contamination of the wound. Fluid loss may be extensive and shock may ensue.

In evaluating burns in the adult victim, the rescuer may have a reasonably accurate estimate of the body surface area that is involved using the rule of nines (See Figure 13 for percent of body surface burned). Each arm is estimated as nine percent of body surface area, each leg is eighteen percent, the back and buttocks are eighteen percent, and the head and neck are nine percent. The larger the involved body area, the lower the likelihood of survival.

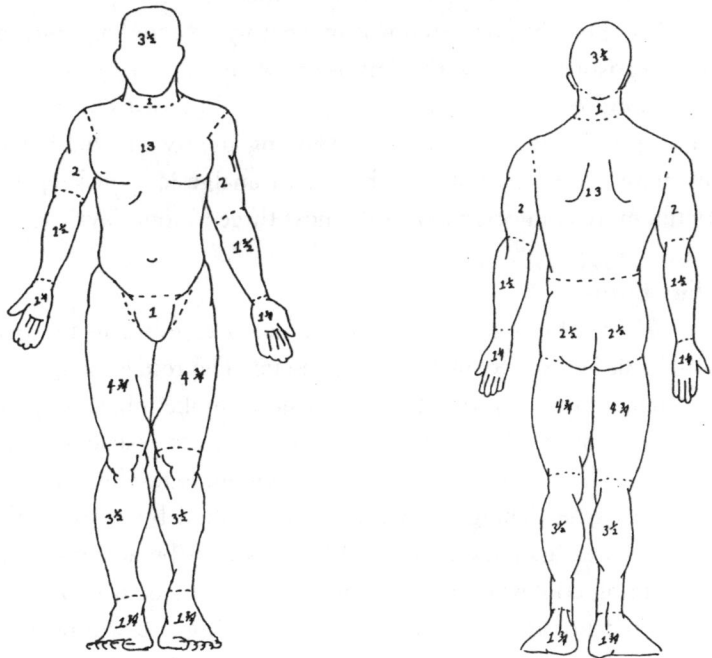

Figure 13 Percent of total body surface area involved in burns.

•Sunburn

Solar radiation can inflict a serious and painful burn in a short time. Everyone can benefit from sunscreen. People of all races and skin color will reduce the likelihood of serious sunburns during prolonged sun exposure. The ultraviolet rays that cause burns penetrate clouds and therefore sunscreen will be indicated, even on overcast skies. The top of the head, the top of the ears, the back of the shoulders, and the top of the feet are frequently ignored areas that will feel the effects of the sun. Divers should be sure to use waterproof sunscreen. The higher the SPF (sun protection factor) rating, the more protected the diver will be. Often the lure of getting that "great tan" can ruin a dive trip. You can't support a vest and tank on a burned back, and you won't be able to tolerate the pressure of a mask on a burned face. Most sunburns may be classified as first degree burns from radiation exposure.

If sunburn has occurred it is mandatory to avoid any further sun exposure, even with sunscreen. Application of an aloe-containing cream with moisturizer and cold moist compresses will help alleviate discomfort. Drinking plenty of liquids will maintain proper hydration. The use of analgesics will keep the victim more comfortable over the next three to four days.

•Fire Burns

When a fire occurs, the rescuer needs to evaluate the personal risk before attempting a fire rescue. The rescuer may need to balance the risks from heat, explosion, smoke inhalation, and structural failures before venturing into a fire to rescue any victims. The first order of care of a burn victim is to eliminate any further tissue damage. This is accomplished by cooling the affected area as quickly as possible. This may be accomplished by pouring cool water over the area until the tissue is cool. Care is needed not to overcool a victim. Dousing the wound with water may not be wise around the mouth area. Burns of the face and chest may cause breathing difficulty. Smoke inhalation may further complicate fire injuries, leading to serious lung impairment. The majority of fire victims succumb to smoke inhalation and not to the burns from the fire itself. Oxygen therapy may be indicated but the use of oxygen in a fire environment must be cautiously evaluated.

Shock may be an associated complication of a burn victim. The deeper burns may be involved with significant fluid loss. Large areas on small victims are especially dangerous because of rapid loss of fluid leading to shock. The burned tissue on a wound (eschar) should not be removed. This eschar may help limit fluid loss and contamination of the wound in the field. Avoid contamination of the affected area by cutting away clothing, washing the wound with sterile water if possible, and applying a sterile dressing.

•Hot Liquids

Hot liquid burns fall into the same classifications but the depth of injury may not be so readily obvious. The skin remains intact in most instances during the initial injury. Cooling the area is of utmost importance by pouring cold water over the area for at least ten minutes. A burn cream may be of assistance. A sterile dressing is applied.

•Chemical Burns

Acids and alkaline solutions are the usual causes of chemical burns. Although both can cause serious injury, acids usually produce more superficial damage while alkaline solutions produce deeper and more serious injury. Chemical burns demand cutting away clothing that may also be contaminated by the offending chemical. The rescuer must take care to avoid injury to himself or herself or further injury to the victim, especially the eyes or mouth from contaminated clothing. Inhalation of acidic or alkaline fumes must be avoided as it may lead to serious bronchial or pulmonary damage. Flooding the affected area with continuous water to dilute and wash away the chemical is the best management in the field. Flushing out of the area is continued until help arrives, if possible. A minimum of ten minutes of irrigating the wound or affected area is recommended for minor exposures. Application of an antibiotic ointment and covering the area with sterile gauze may be indicated until medical attention is sought.

•Electrical Burns

Electrical fires, especially on a boat, can be extremely hazardous. Approaching a victim of electric injuries may be risky for the rescuers. The first order of concern is to be sure circuits are shut off and electrical current has been eliminated. Once the rescuer and victim are out of electrical or fire danger the victim is thoroughly assessed.

There are three different types of burns incurred by electricity. First is the injury received from the thermal injury. These are to be classified and treated as other burns. The entrance and exit sites of the electrical current may be quite deep. Fire can occur at the entrance or exit site on the skin, clothing, or surrounding structures. These fire-related burns are also classified and treated as other burns. The damage caused by the current flow through the body may be invisible but the most serious. If the current passes through the heart or brainstem the victim dies immediately. If the current passes through the muscles the damage releases proteins that can cause kidney failure. The contractions of the muscle can cause fractures. The victim should therefore be evaluated for deformities or tenderness that may indicate a fracture of the long bones and then be treated with the proper splints and evaluation of the pulses. All thermal burn sites are to be cooled with water. The charred areas are not to be removed in the field, but instead should be covered with a burn cream or antibiotic ointment and dressed with sterile gauze.

Monitoring vital signs is continued as respiratory and cardiac arrest may require CPR. Seizure management may be needed as well.

- **Rope or Friction**

These burns are classified by the depth of tissue that has been rubbed off or the depth of the heat damage produced. They are treated in the same manner as a comparable thermal injury. Fractures or stretch and twisting type injures may accompany these injuries. Splinting and careful observation for swelling and bleeding may be required. Raising the affected area and immobilizing the neck for a whiplash injury may be indicated.

Hypothermia

Hypothermia is defined as core body temperature below normal. This is usually considered to be below 97 degrees Fahrenheit (about 36.1 degrees Celsius). The body may lose heat from water, air, or a combination of these. As water evaporates off the body surface, it robs the body of heat energy to convert the water to water vapor. This is an important source of heat loss for divers after a dive when they have already lost body heat during the dive. It is wise to dry off as quickly as possible after a dive to prevent further cooling.

A diver will experience heat loss twenty times faster in water than in air. This is why even in warm water a diver will need insulation during repetitive dives. Up to 50% to 75% of a person's heat loss can occur from the head either during diving or in cold weather. The use of a hood can decrease this heat loss during a dive, and the use of a hat may substantially decrease heat loss in cold weather. Much of the heat that is calculated to be lost from the head is in the form of warm humidity during breathing. It is known that rebreathing systems can significantly decrease this loss because the air that is recirculated is already warmed.

Shivering, confusion, altered mental status, or fatigue are common early symptoms of hypothermia. Rigidity followed by total muscular relaxation, bradycardia (slow heart rate), loss of consciousness, slowed respirations, and cardiac arrhythmias (abnormal heart rate) are signs of advanced hypothermia. If a diver is experiencing the early symptoms, the dive should be terminated and wet clothing removed. The diver should get out of the wind, and use several layers of warm clothing and covers to protect himself or herself from any further heat loss. The diver may benefit from intake of warm beverages.

The person in hypothermia can be warmed with moist or dry heat. Intake of warm fluids greatly increases core temperature. Care must be taken not to put anything into the mouth of an individual with an altered mental status. They may aspirate (inhale) rather than swallow the drink. Body warmth is a good source of heat and laying next to a person with hypothermia may accelerate rewarming if there is no other source of heat. Monitoring core body temperature may be done, especially in a victim with an altered mental status, to evaluate the progression and effectiveness of rewarming.

Hyperthermia

The inability of the body to rid itself of heat may lead to hyperthermia (overheating). The body can tolerate temperatures up to about 103 degrees Fahrenheit (39.4 degrees C). Beyond that, chemical alterations in the body begin to interfere with normal physiology. There is a continuum from heat exhaustion that may progress to heatstroke. Exercise-induced heatstroke and exhaustion usually affect young victims whereas sedentary heatstroke and exhaustion affects elderly or overweight individuals. In this condition the cardiovascular system is unable to adapt to a hot environment. The diver may suffer from hyperthermia before, between, and after dives from thick exposure suits that are worn in hot weather in preparation for cold water diving. In a tropical climate the diver may become hyperthermic from exposure to hot weather or sunshine without shade. Maintaining good hydration with cool beverages and staying in a shaded area may help prevent becoming overheated. Donning wet or dry suits just before entry and either removing or partially removing the suits between dives is recommended.

Heat Exhaustion

Heat exhaustion tends to affect those who become dehydrated in a hot environment. The victim may feel dizzy, weak, and have a headache. They feel moist and clammy. They look pale and sweaty. The pulse is weak and rapid. They should lie flat in a cool place and drink plenty of cool beverages. Elevating the feet above the heart may help the victim feel better. Cooling the body may be done with water or wet towels. Unrecognized or untreated, heat exhaustion may progress to heat stroke. Heat cramps can be associated with both conditions. The severe muscular contractions can produce muscle and kidney damage. Medical attention may be required if the condition progresses and the victim cannot be cooled.

Heat Stroke

Failure of the body's heat regulating abilities is termed heat stroke. The victim will experience dizziness, loss of coordination, confusion, and disorientation. Untreated, the victim may become comatose and experience seizures. The skin is flushed and red with no sweat. The skin feels hot and dry. The temperature usually is above 105 degrees Fahrenheit (40.6 degrees C). Irreversible heart and brain damage can occur if the temperature is not quickly lowered.

Cooling the victim as soon as possible is imperative. If the victim is conscious cool water or beverages may be given. Cooling the body with continuous bathing of cold water or ice will rapidly decrease the core body temperature. An alcohol sponge bath may also help cool the body. Take care not to overcool the core temperature. Rectal temperatures are the most reliable for monitoring core temperatures. Monitoring the vital signs is very important. CPR or management of convulsions may be required.

Seasickness

Seasickness is caused by the discrepancy of the information reaching the brain from the visual and vestibular systems. This usually occurs when an individual is inside a moving vehicle or vessel and the eyes are fixed on objects within the vehicle or vessel. The vestibular system within the inner ear senses the motion that is out of sync with the visual information being sent to the brain. Being within the cabin of a rocking or moving vessel, reading while swaying, and inhaling automotive fumes may all worsen symptoms of seasickness.

Riding on deck or gazing out a window so that the individual can visualize the swaying that the vestibular system is sensing helps prevent seasickness. Refraining from activities where the individual is focusing on objects that are also swaying such as reading, or working within the cabin of a vessel will help. Staying away from the stern of the vessel where the fumes rise will help to prevent seasickness.

A multitude of medications is available to help prevent seasickness. These medications are best taken before the individual boards the vessel, or at least before the symptoms of seasickness begin. Taking these medications after the symptoms of seasickness begin rarely resolves or improves the condition. Either patches or tablets may deliver these medications. The diver may prefer tablets to prevent the patch from falling off during the dive. Side effects may be a consideration for the diver. Checking the product information sheets that come with the medication will inform the diver of potential undesirable side effects. The patches are to be handled carefully because the drugs used can cause dilatation of the pupils if the user rubs his or her eyes after handling the patches. This will lead to blurred vision in the affected eye for a considerable period of time. Bracelets are also available that press on specific pressure points on the wrist to prevent seasickness. Variable results, usually disappointing, may be expected from these bracelets.

If a passenger does suffer from seasickness, they should not be given food. It is a misconception that food helps. It is also a common habit to have the victim lock himself or herself in the head to vomit in privacy. The enclosed room will propagate the symptoms. The victims should avoid the cabin altogether. Staying out in the open air, looking at the horizon, and standing away from the engine fumes is recommended. If anchored or moored, they may take a swim or get on a raft to get off the boat. Although the raft will also sway, the proximity to the water surface may help.

When a passenger is sick they may be directed to the edge of the vessel to avoid soiling the deck. When moored or anchored, the passenger may be directed to the leeward side of the bow where the hull slants back the most. If underway, they may be directed to the leeward side at the stern. Other passengers should be kept away as the sight and smell of someone vomiting can cause a chain reaction amongst the others. Any mess on deck should therefore be cleaned immediately. Having victims gargle or rinse out their mouth may eliminate the distaste and help them feel better.

Fractures

Skull Fractures

Skull fractures may be caused from blunt or penetrating head injuries. Penetrating injuries are usually readily diagnosable whereas blunt injuries may produce fractures that are not so easily discernable. Inspection of the head for swelling, bleeding, and discoloration may reveal areas of injury. Feeling the scalp on all surfaces may reveal indentations that indicate a depressed skull fracture. The skull ordinarily has several indentations and ridges and is for the most part symmetrical with the opposite side. Comparison with the two sides is important to determine if the indentation may be a true injury or just part of the individual's anatomy. If a spinal injury is suspected, inspection of the head should be done with the head and neck immobilized.

The rescuer should inspect every orifice on the head for signs of injury. The ear canals, the eyes, the nostrils, and the mouth need to be visually examined. Bleeding or drainage of clear fluid from any of these orifices would indicate a potentially serious problem. Bleeding would indicate a deeper injury than just a surface wound. Leakage of clear fluid would indicate a basilar skull fracture with leakage of cerebrospinal fluid. Many times the cerebrospinal fluid may leak mixed with blood. A clear ring around a central bloodstain on a cloth would indicate the presence of cerebrospinal fluid (the "ring sign"). The association with serious brain injuries or the potential for a brain infection is quite high with these injuries and medical attention is warranted as soon as possible.

Inspection of the skin around the face and scalp may give clues about deeper injuries. Bruising around the eye, especially if involving the areas around both eyes (Raccoon sign) is indicative of a frontal basilar skull fracture. Bruising over the mastoid process located behind and below the ear (Battle sign) is indicative of a temporal or occipital basilar skull fracture. Both of these fractures may be associated with leakage of cerebrospinal fluid. The frontal basilar skull fracture may cause leakage of cerebrospinal fluid from the nose whereas the temporal basilar skull fracture may cause cerebrospinal fluid leakage from the ear.

Blunt injuries to the head may be associated with serious neck injuries or fractures. Skull fractures may be linear, depressed, or associated with an overlying laceration. Victims may initially be without complaints but delayed deterioration can occur rapidly. A visible or palpable indentation of the skull may alert the rescuer of the likelihood of a depressed skull fracture. The lack of a depression on the scalp is no assurance that there is no depression of a fracture since blood collected under the scalp may fill in and conceal the depression.

Skull fractures have a high incidence of bleeding inside the skull (epidural hematoma, subdural hematoma, or intracerebral hematoma). These may all be surgical emergencies and need to be evaluated in a hospital setting. Significant bleeding inside the skull may cause an increase in intracranial pressure (pressure inside the skull). A patient may go into a coma and require CPR. If increased pressure on the brain from bleeding is suspected, rescue breathing should be done twice as frequently as otherwise would be given in an attempt to decrease the intracranial pressure. This should be done with two or three rescuers alternating rescue breathing since a single rescuer will not be able to maintain this rate of rescue breathing for very long. Twenty-five to thirty-five breaths per minute will bring about reduction of intracranial pressure that may benefit a victim with intracranial bleeding.

Seizures may be associated with these injuries and proper seizure management should be followed. Lacerations and abrasions need to be carefully evaluated. Bleeding from a head wound may be more complicated than elsewhere in the body.

Applying direct pressure on a head wound could push a loose bone fragment deeper into the brain or cause an increase in intracranial pressure. Bleeding from the head may be from the scalp or from deeper tissues. Direct pressure on a bleeding head wound may also direct the flow of blood into the brain instead of allowing the blood to drain out of the wound. Scalp bleeding may be controlled by compressing pressure points just anterior and above the ear canal (superficial temporal artery) or from pressure points about one to three inches on either side of the midline on the back of the head (occipital arteries). Direct pressure on the carotid arteries on either side of the trachea should never be used to stop bleeding in the field. Placing loose gauze over the bleeding area may encourage clot formation and stop bleeding.

Spine Fractures

Fractures of the spine are frequently associated with other major or minor injuries of the head, chest, abdomen, or extremities. The victim may or may not exhibit symptoms of a spinal fracture with neurological deficit. The major neurological symptoms may include pain of the injured area, numbness, weakness, paralysis, difficulty or lack of breathing, or blood pressure changes. Changes in heart rate may also accompany a spinal cord injury. Injuries to the spinal cord may be associated with displacement of an intervertebral disc without a spinal fracture, but must be treated as cautiously as a spinal fracture due to the possibility of irreversible nerve root or spinal cord injury.

Severe occipital headache and tenderness may be associated with fractures of the first cervical vertebra, the Atlas. The victims routinely are unable to flex their head and frequently need to hold their head up by the chin with their hand. Severe pain or inability to rotate the head after a diving injury where the victim struck the head on entry is indicative of a fracture of the second cervical vertebra, the Axis. This injury is life threatening. Both of these injuries require immediate firm immobilization.

Fractures of the tailbone (coccyx) are associated with a fall into the sitting position. Severe jolts and bounces during a rough boat ride while sitting on a hard surface can produce the same injury. Severe tenderness of the tailbone is the hallmark sign. The victim should lay facedown to avoid pressure and movement of the fractured bone fragment. Numbness around the anus may accompany this injury if the nerves are injured.

The best management of a suspected spinal injury in the field is immobilization of the entire spine until professional assistance arrives. This can be accomplished by laying the victim with the spine in a straight manner. Assigning a rescuer to hold the head straight and keep the victim from moving is the best method to achieve this goal. Laying the victim on a plank or door will allow for moving the victim if need-be without altering the position of the spine. If there is no available board the victim should be maintained without movement. If moving them is inevitable four rescuers need to straddle the victim and a fifth rescuer is assigned to hold the head straight, cradling the head on their forearms (See Figure 17 for Five rescuers carrying spine victim). Lifting and moving the victim is done with one rescuer (preferably the one at the head) coordinating moves so that it is done simultaneously without altering the position of the entire spine. The neck can also be immobilized by placing a newspaper or magazine behind the victim's head, wrapping it behind the head, and taping it to their forehead. It can also be done with anything available to be placed on either side of the head while the person lies on their back. A person solely dedicated to manually immobilizing the head is the best method for the comatose or the alert victim. Frequent checks of the vital signs and neurological status is important, all the while not allowing movement of the spine.

Should the victim begin to vomit, they can be rolled into a three-quarter prone position (See Figure 14 for Three-Quarter

Prone Position). The victim is rolled onto one side and has the arm on the ground extended above the head so that it can lie on the bicep muscle. The other arm is bent and placed so that the elbow is supported on the ground. The leg on the ground is kept straight while the other is bent at the hip and knee so the knee is supported on the ground. The victim is rolled so the chest forms about a forty-five degree angle with the ground. The victim's face is also facing downward about forty-five degrees. The spine is maintained straight and will allow vomitus to flow out of the mouth and reduce the risk of aspiration.

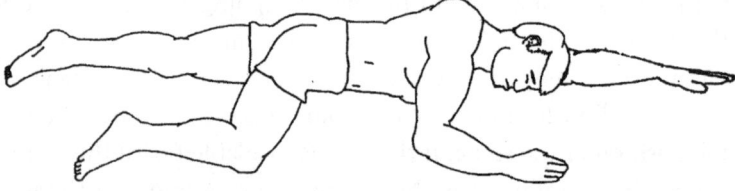

Figure 14 Three-quarter prone position

A sole rescuer with a spine injury victim who must be moved out of harm's way may find a board and slide it under the victim. In order to get the board under the victim, the sole rescuer can roll the victim into a three-quarter prone position while attempting to maintain the spine as straight as possible. The board is then placed behind the victim and the victim is gently and carefully rolled back onto the board. The victim is centered on the board and secured. A cloth, strap, or tape may be used to secure the victim's forehead to the board to keep the head straight while lifting the board at the head end and dragging the victim out (See Figure 15 for Single rescuer moving spine victim). Two rescuers may do the same with more ease. When two rescuers are involved, the board may be easily lifted at both ends and carried (See Figure 16 for Two rescuers carrying spine victim). A sole rescuer may use a board, two paddles, a shelf, or a cabinet door. Many other objects may be substituted if a board is not available.

MEDICAL MANAGEMENT

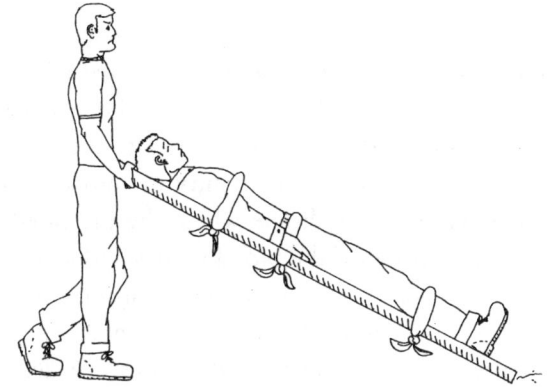

Figure 15 Single rescuer carrying a spine victim on board.

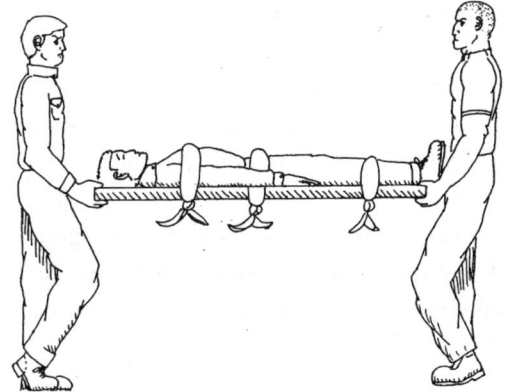

Figure 16 Two rescuers carrying a spine victim on board.

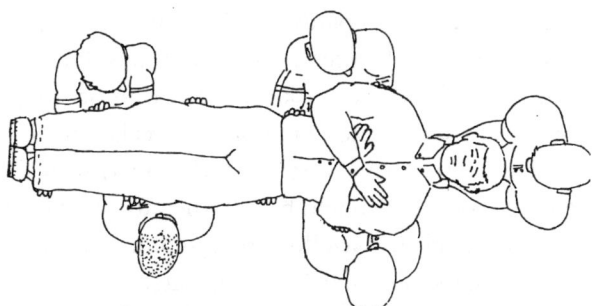

Figure 17 Five rescuers carrying a spine victim.

Extremity Fractures

Fractures of the extremities may be non-displaced, displaced, or compound. These fractures may be associated with extensive soft tissue damage. Injury to the nerves may lead to loss of sensation or movement distal to the fracture. Injuries to the blood vessels may cause bleeding from the extremity or into the extremity, causing a compartment syndrome where the increased pressure can lead to compression of the blood vessels and lack of circulation to the distal aspect of the extremity. This may be a surgical emergency that could result in loss of the limb. On occasion, a fracture of the long bones in the extremities may lead to a fat embolus that can cause lack of circulation to the lungs and in severe cases may lead to respiratory distress and death.

Careful inspection of the injured limb may reveal distortion of the extremity, discoloration, swelling, or loss of sensation, movement, or pulses. The management of suspected fractures should include immobilization and splinting. Application of ice and elevation of the limb above the victim's heart may help decrease the swelling of the affected area. Ongoing monitoring of the limb for sensation, movement distal to the fracture, and pulses should be continued. Immediate attention by medical personnel is indicated.

Splints may be made from a variety of common items. Newspapers, magazines, or cardboard may be wrapped around the extremity and taped. Boards, paddles, pillows, fins, and many other objects may also be used as substitutes to splint the extremity. The rule to follow is to make sure the tape or string around the splints is not so tight to compromise circulation to the distal areas of the extremity. The area of the fracture should be covered with ice but should be left open to allow for frequent inspection to check for swelling or discoloration. Extremities that are distorted should not be manipulated by untrained individuals, but instead should be immobilized as they are. Nerve or blood vessel damage can be caused by attempting to reduce displaced fractures in the field by untrained personnel. If there is a lack of pulses in an extremity due to a severely distorted fracture, the rescuer may attempt to establish anatomical positioning of the limb in order to re-establish blood flow to the limb. The limb is then to be immobilized with a splint.

Concussion

Coma vs. Concussion

Head injuries can occur due to rough weather, a tank or diver falling onto a diver below, being struck by a boat, or many other causes. A temporary loss of consciousness or a temporary lapse of normal neurological function (imbalance, speech problems, amnesia, etc.) would be termed a concussion. If the victim does not regain consciousness despite stimulation after a few minutes they may be in a coma (a prolonged and sustained state of unconsciousness). Both injuries are serious and need to be evaluated by a medical professional as soon as possible. Coma after a head injury is due to bleeding within the skull until proven otherwise by a CAT scan. The coma is almost always due to an increase in pressure within the skull (increased intracranial pressure) that restricts blood flow to the brain. There is a high death rate for these injuries despite all efforts. Timely evacuation of the blood clot and control of bleeding is the only hope of altering the inevitable progression to death. Many head injuries are associated with neck and facial injuries. Treating the unconscious victim as a potential neck injury victim will protect all victims until radiologically confirmed to have no cervical fracture.

The initial management of an individual who has lost consciousness is to maintain an open **A**irway, ensure that **B**reathing continues, and check that the victim has adequate blood **C**irculation. These are the **ABC**'s of emergency evaluations of victims. If any of these are in doubt, then CPR is to be given. Victims with suspected bleeding in the skull may benefit from being hyperventilated (faster than normal breathing, see above). Immobilization of the neck is achieved and a quick over-all assessment is conducted of the victim's body looking for any and all bruises, swelling, punctures, lacerations, discoloration, and deformities. A second rescuer may attend to the proper management of other wounds.

If the victim regains consciousness, they are to remain still. A better evaluation of associated injuries can be done with a conscious victim. Areas of pain, tenderness, and weakness or paralysis can be established. Frequent evaluations of pulse, breathing, orientation, and communication are monitored until medical professionals arrive.

Convulsions

Commonly referred to as seizures or epileptic fits, these attacks can be quite dramatic. They are caused by uncontrolled waves of electrical discharges in the brain. Many circumstances may cause a seizure. Lack of oxygen (anoxia), oxygen toxicity, head injuries, hyperthermia (overheating), medication side effects, and toxins are commonly encountered dive-related causes.

There are many types of seizures, but the most common is the generalized tonic-clonic seizure. The victim may have a sense of uneasiness or aura just before the attack. Most auras consist of a peculiar sensation or smell immediately before the event. The victim then either loses all muscular tone or becomes rigid and collapses. The body begins to have rhythmic, usually rapid alternating movements. The movement may be generalized, involving the entire body from the start, or begin with one part of the body and slowly or rapidly spread to the rest of the body.

Seizures routinely last a few seconds before the victim calms down and enters a period of unresponsiveness that usually lasts several minutes. At times seizures may be prolonged or follow each other in rapid sequence. This is referred to as status epilepticus. This may be a dangerous event since respirations may be halted due to the sustained contractions of the muscles of respiration. The excessive production of lactic acid from the continued forceful contractions may lead to a metabolic acidosis that could affect the heart.

Management in the field should be limited to preventing secondary injuries and calling for help. If victims begin to experience peculiar sensations or sensing smells that are not present, they should be asked to lie down. Asking them to sit down is not recommended if anticipating a seizure. When the muscular contractions begin, keep objects away from victims to prevent injury. One may place a pillow under their head to pad the head from striking the floor. Do not try to place anything in their mouth. This could be dangerous for the victim and the rescuer.

After the muscular contractions have stopped and the victim is unresponsive, attention to airway preservation is the first priority. If the victim has bitten their tongue and is bleeding, place the victim in the three-quarter prone position to prevent the blood from being aspirated. Pressure may be applied on the tongue by rolling gauze around it only after the victim is awake enough not to bite the rescuer. After the victim has regained consciousness, do not allow the victim to get up since repeated seizures are common. After experiencing a seizure, victims are frequently disoriented and confused. Keep them comfortable and on the ground and reassure them you are taking care of them. Continue to monitor the victim's vital signs and attend to any injuries that occurred during the seizure or that preceded the seizure until paramedics arrive.

Amputation

Amputations can occur from propeller injuries, shark attacks, alligator/crocodile attacks, as well as bites from eels, barracudas, and other animals. Rescuing a diver may be difficult and care must be taken that the rescuer does not endanger himself or herself in the process. Amputations can appear quite dramatic and affect the rescuer in a variety of ways. Squeamish individuals and children should be removed from the area to avoid long term psychological trauma or to prevent someone from passing out and possibly sustaining an injury of their own.

The rescuers should use appropriate barriers (masks, gloves, and eye shields) when dealing with these wounds. Significant blood loss can occur in a very short time. The primary concern of the rescuer should be to limit blood loss and prevent or treat shock as quickly as possible. The amputated body part, if salvaged, should be kept on ice but not allowed to freeze for possible re-attachment. If the body part is still attached by a minimal amount of tissue, it should be splinted in place in the most proper anatomical position and also wrapped with ice.

The most effective method of stopping blood loss in this case is with a tourniquet (See Figure 18 for Application of Tourniquet). The tourniquet should be placed as close to the injury as possible to limit further tissue injury. Amputations may be associated with a clean cut or may be associated with rotation and tearing of the limb. Clean-cut injuries allow for the tourniquet to be placed near the end of the stump. The injuries associated with rotation and tearing of tissues may have tissue damage that extends well into the remaining extremity stump. These injuries may require a tourniquet much more proximal on the limb to control bleeding, or application of pressure on a major artery at a pressure point well above the amputation.

In particular cases, direct pressure may control the bleeding, especially where there is no stump to place a tourniquet.

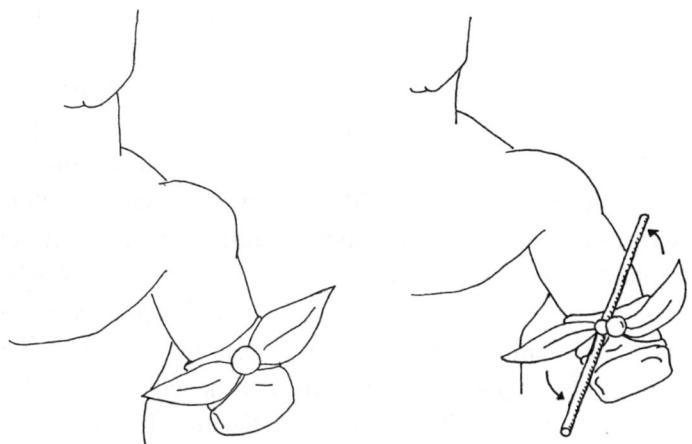

Figure 18 Application of Tourniquet.

Tying off the major blood vessels (artery and vein) with thread, string, or suture can be done. The rescuer should clamp the vessel with a hemostat and then double tie the vessel before removing the hemostat. Use of a clamp or snap (hemostat) can also accomplish the same thing without tying off of the vessel, although applying a dressing over a clamp or snap may be more difficult. Placing a sterile dressing on the wound will help prevent infection and induce hemostasis (to stop bleeding) until medical help arrives.

Hemorrhage

Whenever caring for a bleeding victim the rescuer should use a protective barrier such as gloves, goggles, eye shield, mask, etc. All debris produced by the treatment of a bleeding wound should be disposed of in a plastic bag, preferably with an appropriate label. This should be saved for future reference if needed. Blood-soaked gauze and clothing should be saved because an estimate of the victim's blood loss may be obtained from them.

Limiting blood loss should be done with direct pressure if the blood loss involves the chest, abdomen, or head. Care is taken to not displace broken bone fragments that can puncture the lung (rib fracture) or be pushed into the brain (skull fracture). Blood loss from an extremity can also be quickly and effectively controlled with pressure over the artery proximal to the bleeding site. These areas are called pressure points. These areas where feeding arteries run are behind the knees, at the inguinal area on either side of the groin, the radial artery at the wrist, the inside of the elbow, and the axilla (armpit) (See Figure 1 for Location of Pulses. Pressure points are in the same locations in addition to the others listed).

Tourniquets can be very effective tools for controlling blood loss, but may cause extensive tissue necrosis due to lack of blood flow and should be used only as a last resort. The wider the tourniquet, the less tissue damage is caused by the tourniquet itself. If used for the proper indication and length of time, they can be useful for stopping blood loss. For instance, when one rescuer is trying to bring a bleeding diver or swimmer in, a temporary tourniquet may facilitate preventing blood loss during the rescue. Tourniquets should only be tight enough to stop the bleeding. Over time, it may be possible to release the tourniquet slowly without initiating blood loss or loosened with concomitant direct pressure over the bleeding site to control bleeding. Tourniquets may be released every 30 to 120 seconds to perfuse the extremity and check if the bleeding has stopped. If only minimal oozing persists, direct pressure alone may then control the bleeding. A tourniquet is the preferred means of stopping the bleeding from an amputated extremity (such as from either a shark attack or propeller injury). A tourniquet is not to be released at all if being used for an amputation. The tourniquet needs to be placed as close to the bleeding point as possible to limit tissue damage.

To apply a tourniquet the rescuer may preferably use a handkerchief or piece of cloth (but rope, string or other strap may be used) (See Figure 18 for Application of Tourniquet). The tourniquet material is wrapped around the extremity and one or two knots are made. A stick or tool is laid over the knot and another knot is made over the stick. The stick is then turned to tighten the tourniquet only to the point where the blood stops or is controllable with pressure. The stick is then secured in that position by holding it there, or another knot is made holding the end of the stick from turning back.

If the victim is bleeding from an amputated extremity where there is no stump, such as from the shoulder or hip, there may be no pressure point above the area of bleeding. Firm direct pressure may be attempted. If bleeding is still significant and uncontrolled, the rescuer may need to find and clamp the vessels directly to save the victim's life. Bleeding occurs from the artery and the vein and both need to be clamped or tied off. The rescuer must be able to visualize the vessel in order to apply the hemostat or clamp accurately. The best method of achieving this is to apply gauze to the wound with firm pressure to slow down the bleeding. Slowly roll the gauze away starting on one side toward the other while maintaining firm pressure. As the open ends of vessels are uncovered they can be seen to begin bleeding. Hemostats or clamps should they be applied across the vessel, trying to leave a cuff of vessel beyond the hemostat so that it does not slip off. If the rescuer has only one clamp the vessel can be tied off with suture, string, thread, or whatever material is available. The vessel should be double or triple tied to ensure the knot will not open or the tie slip off. The clamp can then be removed and the gauze further rolled away to clamp other lacerated vessels. Only the major vessels need to be tied or clamped. Smaller vessels should be able to be controlled with direct pressure.

If a diver encounters a significant injury to an extremity while diving and is having significant blood loss, direct pressure may control the hemorrhaging. Formation of a surface blood clot is unlikely to occur while underwater because of the continuous washing off of the blood from the wound. Bleeding at depth may be difficult to perceive since blood appears black or gray at depth. The volume of blood lost may be difficult to assess because the blood is washed away immediately. A tourniquet can be useful in water until the diver is out of the water. A tourniquet can be fashioned underwater out of the strap of a dive tool sheath or a retractable line. Penetrating injuries with a foreign object still imbedded in the diver should be left in place until the diver is brought to the surface. Removing a spear or piece of imbedded material can initiate uncontrolled bleeding from a lacerated blood vessel that may have been compressed by the object.

Drowning

Drowning occurs when an individual dies due to aspiration of water. Near drowning is when the individual is revived. The damage to the lungs that occurs from water can lead to serious difficulties in the gas exchange function of the lungs and can lead to death. This is known as secondary drowning. There may be many causes of drowning or aspiration. Aspiration of water can cause an individual to cough and choke. If the individual is underwater or at the surface, the coughing and choking can produce repeated aspirations. The rescuer must be attentive to associated injuries or precipitating causes of a drowning victim. A thorough survey of the victim should be completed in an expeditious manner while resuscitation is initiated. A victim who has had rescue breathing begun while in tow or in the water should have rescue breathing interrupted for the shortest period of time possible while the victim is being taken out of the water and onto a boat or shore.

The drowning victim should have the lungs emptied of water being turned face down and having the chest firmly squeezed. Rescue breathing will reexpand the lungs with air. Even if there is water still left in the lungs the alveoli (small air pockets in the lungs) will reexpand with rescue breathing and have some surface area exposed to air for gas exchange to occur. A pocket mask with an oxygen connection port will assist in delivery of high oxygen concentrations during rescue breathing.

If the level of consciousness is decreased in an aspiration victim, they must be evaluated with frequent checks of their pulse and respiratory rate. Oxygen is given. If the rate or depth of breathing is diminished, rescue breathing is to be started. If the lungs have been affected significantly the victim may have a very rapid respiratory rate initially. Fatigue may cause them to eventually slow their rate of breathing and may then require rescue breathing. Care is taken to prevent aspiration of vomitus, which is very common in this circumstance. Place the victim in the three-quarter prone position until vomiting stops; then clean out the victim's mouth and resume rescue breathing in the supine position (on the back).

If a diver has a significant choking episode from water aspiration but maintains consciousnes, they may be given oxygen and kept warm. Vomiting is a frequent occurrence and care is taken to be sure victims do not aspirate vomitus. Medical attention is sought as soon as possible. Do not give them anything to eat or drink until medical personnel evaluate them. They are not to dive any further that day until cleared by a physician.

A victim who has no pulse or respirations requires full CPR that is continued until medical personnel arrive and take over care. Even completely unresponsive drowning victims have been known to recover with proper attention, especially in cold water environments.

Crush Injury

Crush injuries can occur from heavy objects falling on a body part (such as an air tank) or from being caught between large structures (such as falling between two vessels or between a vessel and the pier). These injuries may cause lacerations, fractures, or injuries to internal organs. These injuries are routinely much more serious than they may initially appear. Prompt medical attention is warranted in all instances of crush injuries.

Chest

Crush injuries to the chest cavity may cause multiple rib fractures, producing a "flail chest" where the victim is unable to effectively inhale due to an area of chest wall that moves independent of the rest of the chest, compromising the bellows effect of the chest cavity. The victim may tolerate small areas of flail chest wall but breathing is quite painful. A large area of chest wall that is flail will require rescue breathing to maintain adequate oxygenation. A collapsed lung (pneumothorax), bleeding into the chest cavity (hemothorax), and a bruise to the heart (cardiac contusion) producing abnormal heart rhythms and ineffective circulation may be associated with these injuries. Tension pneumothorax is seen more commonly with penetrating injuries than with blunt crush injuries but can be seen when a broken rib punctures the lung. Injury can occur to the great vessels (aorta, inferior or superior vena cava) and produce fatal bleeding into the chest cavity and shock.

Victims are to be managed for their injuries as described for pneumothorax and hemothorax as the circumstance dictates. Rescue breathing or CPR may be indicated as well as treatment for shock. There may be associated thoracic spine injuries causing spinal cord injury or the potential for spinal cord damage.

Abdominal

Crush injuries to the abdominal area can produce serious injuries to the internal organs as well as the great vessels and the spine. Considerable internal bleeding can occur without obvious signs until the victim has a drop in blood pressure from the internal loss of blood. Rupture of the intestines can produce a life-threatening sepsis due to spillage of its contents into the abdominal cavity. Injury to the great vessels that course through the abdomen (aorta and inferior vena cava) can cause massive rapid bleeding or an injury to the wall of the artery where the blood dissects into the lining of the wall of the vessel and blocks its flow (dissecting aortic aneurysm). Needless to say, these injuries must be evaluated and treated as soon as possible at a medical facility.

The rescuer should keep a watchful eye on the victim's vital signs (heart rate, blood pressure, respiratory rate, and temperature). Many associated injuries may need attention in the field. The rescuer should make a quick survey of the victim to check their neurological condition that may suggest a spinal injury. Associated fractures of the chest, head, and extremities must be ruled out. Hemorrhaging should be managed in the appropriate manner.

A rescuer may find several signs that suggest internal bleeding. Progressive increase in the abdominal circumference leads to a tense abdominal wall. Discoloration of the skin (either over the belly or at one or both flanks) occurs but may also take time to develop. A weak and rapid pulse is indicative of early hypovolemic shock. Altered mental status (confused or losing consciousness) may develop from decreased blood circulation to the brain from blood loss in the abdomen. Since the rescuer has no possible way of predicting where the bleeding is occurring in the abdomen, specific measures at stopping the blood loss is impossible in the field. Direct pressure on the deep structures of the abdomen is not recommended since this may cause the abdominal structures to push up on the diaphragm and hamper breathing or CPR of the victim. These victims should be closely monitored, and appropriate measures to treat shock and associated injuries, which may include CPR, are given until emergency medical personnel arrive.

Head

Crush injuries of the face and/or head are extremely serious and life threatening. Neck injuries accompany the vast majority of these injuries. Facial and cervical spine injuries may affect the victim's ability to breathe. Massive bleeding, seizures, coma, paralysis, and cardiac and respiratory arrest may all be associated with a high death rate in these victims despite any rescue attempts. Serial neurological exams are indicated to closely monitor the victim.

Rescue attempts should be directed toward stabilization of cervical spine injuries, control of bleeding, and maintenance of the victim's airway and breathing until emergency medical personnel arrive. Cardiac and respiratory arrest may require CPR.

Extremity

Crush injuries to an extremity may result in fractures and soft tissue injuries. Fractures may be quite extensive and may present as compound or comminuted fractures (displaced or protruding bone fragments through the skin). The soft tissue injuries may involve the muscle, ligament or tendons, blood vessels, or nerves. Soft tissue injuries may be a result of the pressure from the injury itself or due to laceration from the broken bone fragments. Extensive deformities, internal or external bleeding, and/or swelling may accompany these injuries.

Management on-site will depend on the specifics of the injury. Bleeding is controlled by the routine prescribed methods. Swelling is managed by elevation and wrapping the extremity with ice. Splinting the extremity is done for immobilization of fractures. Pain may be controlled with analgesics and ice. Avoiding aspirin-containing medications may reduce bleeding. Fractures of the long bones, especially the femur (upper leg bone) may be associated with fat emboli that may block vessels within the lungs and at times cause serious and life-threatening respiratory distress. Severe bleeding into the extremity or tissue swelling may compress the nerves and blood vessels feeding blood to the extremity and lead to paralysis or tissue death beyond the injury site. Monitoring the victim's vital signs, pulses, and neurological status is of vital importance.

Penetrating Injury

Penetrating injuries can occur from missiles, slicing action, or forceful crushing action. Superficial foreign bodies may be removed and the wound cleansed with an antiseptic solution and sterilely dressed. Small deep missiles are to be left in and no attempt should be made at wound exploration and removal in the field. Missiles may have entrance and exit wounds. Quite frequently the exit wound is much larger than the entrance wound with a significant surface area of skin missing or disrupted. Even a very small projectile can cause serious damage if the right anatomical structures are penetrated. If a victim goes down after an explosion, they should be examined for an entrance wound. The entrance wound may appear as a small scratch or abrasion.

Large spear-like missiles that are still in place should be left in place and removed within a medical facility. They should be immobilized as much as possible. If very long or attached to a structure, they may be sawed down but left in place. They may be tamponoding (compressing) a major blood vessel that could bleed uncontrollably if the object is removed.

Chest

Penetrating injuries of the chest cavity may injure the ribs, lungs, heart, or any of the vessels located in the chest. A pneumothorax (collapsed lung) or tension pneumothorax may be commonly encountered. There may also be a hemothorax (bleeding into the chest cavity). The rescuer may need to offer treatment for either of these (See treatment for pneumothorax and hemothorax). An injury that penetrates the heart itself has a very poor prognosis with essentially no chance of survival. Injury to the great vessels within the chest cavity (aorta, inferior vena cava, and superior vena cava) cannot be treated directly in the field, but bleeding into the chest cavity may increase the pressure and require drainage as soon as possible.

If there is a gaping wound that is sucking in air it will need to be covered in an airtight fashion. The best method of re-expanding the lung is to have a rescuer deliver a rescue breath to inflate the lungs. The wound should then be covered with gauze soaked in Vaseline™ or antibiotic ointment in an airtight fashion. The bandage is then covered with dry gauze and tape is applied over the entire dressing. Rescue breathing is required in the majority of penetrating chest injuries due to lung collapse, if not initially, later as the problems within the chest cavity progress. CPR and treatment for shock may be required. Allowing air out through the wound may purge a tension pneumothorax from time to time if the circumstances require.

Abdominal

Penetrating abdominal injuries can involve a multitude of organs either alone or in combination. Massive internal bleeding can occur without obvious initial signs until the victim succumbs to hypovolemic shock. Spillage of intestinal contents may lead to rapid septic shock. Deep lacerations and punctures without a persistent foreign body are best managed with firm direct pressure until paramedics arrive. Penetrating injuries with a foreign body present are best managed with immobilization of the foreign body and supportive care with the victim lying in a horizontal position until paramedics arrive. Vital signs are carefully and frequently monitored and CPR is instituted as needed. Treatment for shock may be instituted as the circumstances require.

Head

Penetrating injuries to the head are quite dramatic and may result in rapid deterioration of the victim. Penetrating injuries to the head many times involve the face or neck and may compound the problem. Neck immobilization should be maintained with all head injuries until the cervical spine has been cleared radiographically in a hospital setting. The penetrating object is not to be removed in the field as it may be compressing lacerated vessels that may bleed uncontrollably if the object is removed. If the object is attached to another structure, it is to be cut close to the victim's head and the victim is to be transported without the embedded object being manipulated.

Penetrating injuries may be due to explosions, spear-gun accidents, falls, vessel collisions, or assaults. If the injury involves the skull there are usually hair and bone fragments routinely encountered within the brain in addition to the missile. Do not attempt to debride the wound in the field. Apply a dressing and provide supportive care until medical personnel arrive. Those injuries that involve only the face and do not penetrate the skull are usually not life-threatening unless they involve the mouth or neck. Although injuries to the eye may leave a victim with a lifelong disability and deformity, they are for the most part not life-threatening unless the injury extends behind the orbit and involves the brain. If a missile has only penetrated the eye, the best management is to cover the eye with a sterile eye patch and get the victim to a medical facility as soon as possible. Do not apply any ointments or solutions to the eye in the field.

Small missiles from an explosion or assault with a handgun may be encountered. High velocity missiles at close range have the potential to penetrate through and through. The entrance wound is usually much smaller than the exit wound. Slow velocity missile encounters may enter and not have the kinetic energy to penetrate the opposite wall of skull. Larger missiles such as spears may completely penetrate from one side to the other because of their weight (momentum), not because of their velocity. Even though the spear gun may appear much more dramatic to a rescuer than a high velocity missile that has passed through the brain, it causes much less damage. This is because high velocity missiles produce a much larger pressure wave that pushes water (brain is 70% water) or air to the side. A high velocity missile can produce a hole passing through the brain many times larger than the missile itself.

Bleeding may be quite profuse if a major vessel has been severed. Facial bleeding can be controlled with direct pressure or packing of the wound followed by direct pressure. Bleeding from the head may be a bit trickier to determine the best management. If the bleeding is from the scalp and the bone beneath is intact, direct pressure may be safe. If on the other hand the bone below is loose or open, direct pressure may cause bleeding to become redirected inward toward the brain or loose bone fragments could be pushed into the brain tissue causing further brain damage. If the source of the bleeding is obvious and accessible, a pair of hemostats may be used to accurately clip the vessel. Two hemostats are usually needed, one on either side of the tear on the vessel. In larger gaping wounds with deep bleeding, the rescuer may elect to lightly apply sterile gauze in the wound and allow the surface area on the cotton to encourage clotting to occur.

If an object is embedded into the face the rescuer may determine if it is best to leave it in place or to remove it. The safest thing to do is to leave it in place. If, however, the object is piercing the thin tissues of the eyelid, cheek, lip, or external ear it may be fairly safe to remove at the scene. Controlling bleeding of these thin tissues after removal of the object is easiest if the rescuer applies pressure on both sides of the thin tissue by pinching the tract of the injury between the fingers. If, however, the object is embedded into deeper facial structures, it is safest to leave the object in place and avoid disturbing it until paramedics arrive. If the embedded object enters the skull it should remain in place undisturbed until the victim is taken to a medical facility.

Brain injuries are frequently associated with neck injuries, seizures, respiratory arrest, shock, and cardiac arrest. Management for these and other associated injuries is continued with the appropriate treatment, including CPR if required until paramedics arrive.

Extremity

Penetrating injuries to the extremities are rarely life threatening except for the potential for massive bleeding, which in most cases should be controllable. A through and through injury with an exit and entrance wound with no residual object is the easiest to manage. Dress the wound with sterile gauze and apply local pressure for bleeding. If the object is still in place (i.e., spear), the initial assessment is to check if the object has damaged nerves or blood vessels. Sensation and pulses are examined beyond the penetration site. If pulses are present, one can feel somewhat confident that the object has not transgressed the artery. If on the other hand the pulses are absent the object may have pierced the artery and fairly brisk bleeding may ensue if the object is removed. It is also possible that the pulse may not be present because of internal bleeding with compression of the artery by the blood clot. Inspection of the puncture site may help differentiate these two possibilities. If the area is soft it is likely the artery has been injured and occluded by the object. If the area is swollen and tense it may be due to a compartment syndrome from venous bleeding causing the lack of pulse, but on the other hand, the swelling may be due to internal bleeding from the injured artery that is lacerated but not completely occluded.

If the foreign body only involves the loose soft tissue it is usually safe to remove and apply pressure to the local area after being properly dressed. Application of an antiseptic and elevation of the extremity would be appropriate. If, however, the foreign body involves the muscle or skeletal structures it is best to leave the object in place and immobilized until medical attention is sought.

Heart Attack

A heart attack is the common term for an acute myocardial infarct. This is a term reserved for when an artery that supplies blood to the heart muscle becomes occluded and a portion of the heart muscle dies. If an area of the heart is receiving less than the required volume of blood flow to maintain normal heart muscle function but there is sufficient blood volume to prevent death of the muscle tissue, the victim may experience chest pain. These symptoms are similar to a heart attack but we refer to this as angina pectoris. This is potentially a reversible problem but may be a warning sign of an impending heart attack.

Heart disease is one of the most common causes of death. The incidence of coronary artery disease is high even in a population we may consider relatively young. Boating may have increased demands on a passenger or crew member from carrying equipment, especially diving gear such as the tanks, and the constant muscular adjustments from a rocking boat skipping over waves. The added stress on the cardiovascular system may come from heat, humidity, and sun exposure. Diving is quite strenuous while donning exposure suits and diving gear.

Maneuvering around while wearing dive gear before getting in the water requires a large amount of energy. Cold water diving is markedly more strenuous than warm water diving. Events underwater can increase tension or anxiety that may raise a diver's heart rate and increase cardiac demand. Encounters with a shark or squeezing through a dark, tight swim-through are just two examples. All of these stresses alone or in combination may be enough to cause a heart attack to an individual who may be at risk.

Symptoms of a heart attack include pain, pressure, squeezing, or heaviness in the chest area, mostly on the left. There may be associated discomfort radiating into the left arm, shoulder, neck, or jaw. The victim may have an uncomfortable sense of impending doom, severe apprehension, lightheadedness, and dizziness. The individual may feel palpitations and a sense of their heart racing. The victim may appear pale and break out in a cold sweat and the pulse may be rapid and at times irregular.

The victim should be placed in a recumbent position with the head slightly elevated. It is recommended that the victim take an aspirin as soon as symptoms appear. High concentrations of oxygen are delivered via a facemask. If the victim takes sublingual nitroglycerine for angina they should take one immediately. If the pulse begins to feel weak, the victim should be laid flat with the legs elevated to treat the cardiogenic shock and help the return of blood to the heart. Close monitoring of the vital signs is extremely important until paramedics arrive. CPR may need to be instituted.

Stroke

A stroke is the common term of an acute cerebral infarct. This occurs when brain tissue is damaged or dies. There are two main types of strokes: hemorrhagic and non-hemorrhagic.

Hemorrhagic stroke occurs when a blood vessel ruptures and bleeding damages brain tissue. There are many causes but the most common are due to high blood pressure and cerebral aneurysms. Hemorrhages from high blood pressure usually (but not always) occur to more elderly individuals whereas aneurysmal hemorrhages can occur at any age, many times during strenuous activity. Non-hemorrhagic stroke is due to occlusion of a blood vessel that feeds blood to the brain. The area of the brain that is fed by the particular vessel that is blocked will die within a few minutes from lack of blood. Causes of non-hemorrhagic strokes are emboli (floating material in the blood) from plaques, fat emboli from broken bones, and air (from decompression illness, pulmonary barotrauma, or other causes).

Symptoms of stroke depend on the type of stroke, the location of the stroke, and the extent of the stroke. Non-hemorrhagic strokes are rarely painful, whereas the hemorrhagic strokes frequently cause the "worst headache of their life." Paralysis, speech difficulty, clumsiness, coma, and death can be associated with either type of stroke. The affected area of brain is usually on the opposite side of the affected body part.

The victims should be laid down with the head slightly elevated. They should be kept warm and high concentrations of oxygen are delivered via a facemask. Nothing should be given by mouth and do not give aspirin to the victims. Close monitoring of the vital signs is continued until paramedics arrive. CPR may need to be instituted.

Shock

In medical terms, shock usually refers to a condition where a victim has lower than normal blood pressure leading to inadequate perfusion of blood to the body's tissues. The drop in blood pressure may be caused by many different factors, either alone or in combination. There are four key elements that determine the level of blood pressure. These are the circulating blood volume, the heart, the blood vessels, and the nervous system. Minor deviations of any of these may be able to be compensated for by the other three and blood pressure may be maintained within a normal range. Major dysfunction or deviations from normal of any one of these elements and the compensatory capacity of the other three will be overcome leading to a drop in blood pressure. The essential organs that must maintain perfusion for survival are the brain, the heart, and the lungs. All other organs may suffer damage if not perfused, but the victim may survive for a more extended period within the field.

The most common signs and symptoms are those of light-headedness, feeling faint, dizziness, nausea, poor coordination, pallor, cold sweat, and loss of consciousness. Depending on the cause of shock, the victim's heartbeat is either very slow or very fast. The pulses are usually weak and thready. Toxins may cause a variety of other symptoms including paralysis, rash, blurred or double vision, and others. Management of shock in the field is directed toward correcting the underlying cause if possible and maintaining circulation to the heart, lungs, and brain.

Hypovolemic Shock

Hypovolemic shock is a drop in blood pressure due to loss of circulating blood volume. The loss of blood volume may be from internal or external bleeding. Severe dehydration or loss of fluid from extensive burns may also lead to lower blood volume and thick, concentrated blood. Controlling blood loss and maintaining proper hydration are the means to preventing hypovolemic shock. If dehydrated, restoring proper hydration with fluid intake is the key to overcoming shock. This may be accomplished with oral or intravenous replacement of fluids. The victim with an altered mental status should never be given anything by mouth. If hyperthermia is a contributing factor to dehydration, this should also be corrected. Remaining recumbent and resting is essential until medical assistance arrives. Elevating the legs and lowering the head will increase cerebral blood flow and may alleviate or lessen the symptoms of shock (See Figure 19 for Position of Shock Victim). High concentrations of oxygen will improve oxygen delivery to the brain even with reduced circulation.

Anaphylactic, Septic, and Toxic Shock

Anaphylactic shock is caused by an allergic reaction that leads to relaxation and dilatation of the blood vessels. Toxic shock is a very similar circumstance where a toxic chemical leads to dilatation of the blood vessels. Septic shock occurs from circulation of bacteria within the blood stream producing dilatation of the peripheral vessels. In all of these conditions the drop in blood pressure occurs because of pooling of blood in the most dependent areas of the body. Severe heat and medication may also cause dilatation of the blood vessels. Blood cannot return to the heart to be pumped out again because the blood is sequestered within enlarged vessels, usually in the legs. Laying the victim on their back and elevating the legs will return the blood within the relaxed

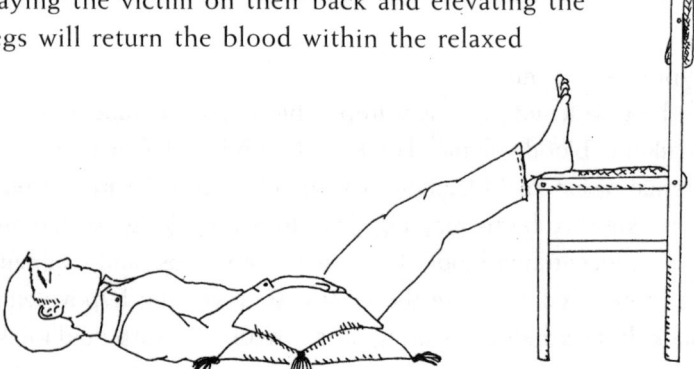

Figure 19 Shock victim with legs elevated on chair and arms elevated on pillows.

blood vessels back to the heart and improve the circulation to the brain (See Figure 19 for Position of Shock Victim). Elevation of the arms will further increase the return of blood to the heart to improve cerebral circulation. Cooling of a heat stroke victim may help the condition and improve survivability. Oxygen therapy is given. If a venomous or toxic injury was the etiological factor that precipitated the condition one may consider isolating the involved injury from the general circulation by application of a tourniquet and ice to further limit venom or toxin absorption.

Cardiogenic Shock

Cardiogenic shock is from failure of the pump (the heart) to circulate the blood from the venous to the arterial side of the circulation. There are many causes of cardiogenic shock. The most common are heart attack, cardiac arrhythmias (abnormal heart rhythm), toxins, compression of the heart (tamponade) by blood or air, and medications. In the case of a heart attack, there may be so much of the heart wall not able to contract that the pumping action is ineffective to maintain blood pressure. Toxins and oxygen derangement could produce heart muscle contractions that are not synchronized (cardiac arrhythmia) and disrupt the pump action of the heart. Increased pressure within the chest cavity (tension pneumothorax, cardiac tamponade, etc.) may reduce or prevent blood from returning to the heart to be pumped out into the circulation. Management is directed toward the specific diagnosis and clinical scenario. Delivery of high oxygen concentrations is indicated regardless of the cause. The victim must be laid on their back with legs elevated (See Figure 19 for Position of Shock Victim). Chest compressions or CPR will artificially replace the pumping action of the heart and may be the most effective treatment for cardiogenic shock in the field until paramedics take over.

Neurogenic Shock

Neurogenic shock is a drop in blood pressure due to an imbalance of nerve stimulation to the heart and/or the blood vessels. The nervous system may cause severe slowing of the heart or relaxation of the blood vessels from a variety of causes including fear, anxiety, spinal cord injury, or head injury. The victim is placed on their back with legs elevated. If the victim is suspected of having a spinal injury, they may be placed on a board to immobilize the spine and tilted in a Trendelenburg position, where the feet are elevated above the level of the head (See Figure 20 for Trendelenburg Position). The diver should be placed in a steep (30 to 60 degrees) position for no more than five or six minutes, if other factors permit this. Prolonging the head down position for more than a few minutes is harmful and will cause cerebral edema. Oxygen is delivered via a facemask. The victim's neurological status and vital signs are closely monitored and CPR may be required to maintain blood circulation.

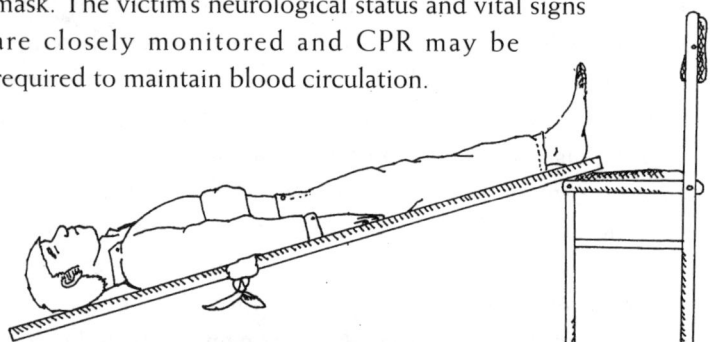

Figure 20 Shock victim with suspected spinal injury immobilized on board in a Trendelenburg position.

Documentation

Documentation of an occurrence or injury serves several purposes. Protection of the rescuers and caregivers is an important legal reason for memorializing an event. Proof that proper protocol was followed is the best protection from liability. More important is that the subsequent caregivers and medical personnel will have a better understanding of the mechanism of injury, the victim's signs and symptoms in the field, and the treatment already delivered. This will give future caregivers the ability to optimize future diagnosis and management of the victim.

Memorializing the event at the time of the occurrence should be done if possible (perhaps by designating a scribe), or if the circumstances won't allow, as soon as possible after the situation has stabilized. Even if the occurrence seemed trivial at the time, it is important to document any event that may resurface in the future as a liability claim. If the passenger or diver refused treatment or attention to the matter, this must also be carefully recorded. Possibly having the individual sign a form that they have refused treatment or help may be seriously considered.

Documentation of an emergency or even a minor injury must begin with recording the time, the location, the witnesses to the occurrence, and the circumstances of the injury. Next note the complaints of the injured individual followed by the observed physical findings on examination. The tentative or working diagnosis may also be documented along with the times of treatment rendered and whatever the response to the treatment was. Efforts at contacting the EMS (Emergency Medical System) and the U.S. Coast Guard or Conservation Police in the area should also be recorded in addition to the response offered by the EMS. The rescuers or those administering first aid need to keep a careful inventory of all tools, instruments, needles, sponges, and all other paraphernalia used and waste generated by an injury. All waste generated during an emergency should be saved for any investigation or insurance carrier to inspect. Photographs, audiotapes, videotapes, specimens, and salvaged items may be of benefit to memorializing the event.

Documentation of pertinent activities for all divers such as boarding times, dive site, entrance and exit times, maximum depth and dive profile, starting and ending tank pressure, buddy assignments, and time of disembarkment may be of vital importance at a later date and should be meticulously recorded. Save all signed waivers together with the records of the dive. Keep all this documentation in a safe place for future reference for at least two years (statute of limitations for civil suits). Keeping the documents off the boat would prevent loss of the records in case of fire or sinking of the vessel.

TABLE 9
DOCUMENTATION

1. Date, day, and time
2. Circumstances leading up to the emergency (boarding times, weather, sea conditions, velocity, location of individuals, etc.)
3. Preserve all dive profile data (dive site, entrance and exit times, starting and ending tank pressure, maximum depth, and buddy)
4. Save liability releases
5. Description of the event
6. Aftermath of the event
7. Individuals involved
8. Witnesses of the event
9. Description of the injuries incurred
10. Complaints and physical findings of the individuals injured
11. Description of the damages incurred
12. Assistance, first aid, or CPR rendered and by whom
13. Response to aid or treatment
14. EMS contacts and their responses
15. Disposition of the victims
16. Any and all pertinent information or descriptions
17. Preserve all pertinent items, videotapes, audiotapes, photos, and specimens

NOTES

CHAPTER FOUR

Underwater Emergencies

Many underwater problems are relatively simple to respond to such as being too cold or inability to clear the ears upon descent. One simply ends the dive and treats the problem as needed. Other problems such as diver injuries, attacks, pulmonary barotrauma, and the unconscious diver may present a much more complicated scenario to contend with. Each circumstance will require a slightly different response, but care of the incapacitated diver should follow certain guidelines. Management of an emergency is always made much easier if more than one rescuer is involved. Rescuers need to take precautions so that they themselves do not become victims as well. If alone, the rescuer should radio for help if possible before attempting the rescue. This may be impossible if the rescuer is the victim's buddy at depth. Assessment of the situation must be accomplished quickly to be sure that the risk/benefit ratio falls heavily on a likely successful outcome before attempting a risky rescue. If the conditions are likely to require more expertise or physical fitness than the rescuer may possess, the rescuer should not attempt the rescue but do whatever he or she can to expedite professional help to be notified quickly. This applies to underwater and surface emergencies alike.

Fatigue

A vast amount of energy is expended preparing for recreational diving. Donning the suit and equipment alone can cause exhaustion. A lengthy boat ride in wavy conditions demands continuous total body muscular adjustments that can also drain a diver before he or she even begins to don the gear. Before even getting to the boat ride, the diver may need to carry a heavy dive bag, weight belt, and one or two tanks to the boat. By the time the diver gets into the water, he or she may already be suffering from early fatigue. The dive itself should be comfortable and leisurely. Fatigue can develop during the dive from swimming against a current, trying to keep up with a quick swimming buddy or group, the effort to move against a thick and stiff wetsuit, a tight vest or suit, heavy work, and undergoing a long surface swim to get to the desired descent location. Hypothermia, shivering, anxiety, and stress can contribute to becoming fatigued. Hyperventilation occurs in response to fatigue, and the more rapid respirations compound the exhaustion of the diver due to the increased work required to move the denser air and the decreased efficiency of rapid breathing.

The only appropriate action is to stop and rest. If you are the diver who is fatigued, notify your buddy and stop. If your buddy is fatigued and wants to rest, you may hold or allow them to hold you if in mid-water (checking your depth gauge frequently to be sure of your buoyancy). It would be easier and more restful if a line or object could be held in order to rest. If your buddy is hyperventilating and you suspect that he or she is fatigued, you should encourage your buddy to stop and rest and to reduce his or her respiratory rate. Signs of hyperventilating may be recognized by more bubbles than usual, seeing the diver clenching the second stage, a rapid respiratory rate, and seeing the diver make exaggerated efforts at breathing (overexpansion of the chest, throwing the head back during each breath, using the neck and shoulder muscles to breath).

Once rested, the divers should proceed in a slower than usual rate. If fatigue recurs the divers should consider terminating the dive. If you are over-weighted and your vest is too tight, you may even consider dropping a few pounds to allow you to deflate the vest in order to loosen it.

Cramps can occur from fatigue amongst other conditions. If cramps occur the diver or buddy may stretch and massage the affected muscle. Rest may be indicated after the cramp has been alleviated before proceeding with the dive to prevent a cramp from recurring. The remainder of the dive should be at a slower and more relaxed pace to prevent further cramping. Repeated cramps may require a dive termination.

Panic

Overreaction to stress may lead a diver to panic. Many situations can precipitate panic reactions including inexperience, enclosed or overhead environments, disorientation, nitrogen narcosis, fatigue, equipment problems, out-of-air situations, or marine animal encounters. Panic may manifest itself with either passive behavior where the diver fails to react and enters a trance–like state, or it can cause the diver to enter an active panic state where the diver overreacts with aggressive or irrational behavior. Either reaction can convert to the other without warning. Both are dangerous situations. A passive panic will prevent the diver from making appropriate buoyancy adjustments which leads to uncontrolled ascents or descents, and the active panic can lead to rapid ascents or wild behavior and potentially cause injury or harm to the diver and/or buddy.

Passive panic should be managed with the buddy cautiously leading the diver to the surface from behind in a slow controlled manner. The rescuer may elect to hold the diver's regulator in their mouth if the need arises. The rescuer should not come within striking distance of the active panic diver but instead attempt to communicate with and calm the victim from a safe distance. The rescuer may attempt to get behind the panic victim and get control of the BCD inflator while firmly holding onto their tank or harness. This will prevent the panic victim from overinflating the BCD and from turning around and causing injury to the rescuer-buddy. The rescuer-buddy can then attempt a controlled and slow ascent. If the panic diver gets away from the rescuer and heads for the surface, the rescuer may try to slow their ascent by grabbing the panic diver's leg and flaring out. This maneuver may cause further panic and intensified struggling on the part of the panic diver. If the diver gets away and ascends too quickly, let go and catch up at the surface.

An out-of-air situation can provoke a panic reaction from one's buddy. The buddy may forcefully pull one's regulator out of one's mouth to breathe. If this occurs do not try to take back the regulator or wrestle for the regulator. Let your buddy take the regulator. One should hold one's buddy close and use one's own alternate air source. Attempts should be made to calm one's buddy and stabilize the situation before attempting a controlled ascent. The proper ascent rate and safety stops must be followed on the way to the surface.

Nitrogen Induced Problems

Nitrogen Narcosis

Silly or bizarre behavior, acting drunk, poor judgement, altered or sloppy diving skills, sleepiness or drowsiness, and poor coordination may be signs of nitrogen narcosis. This condition is related to the effect of nitrogen on the diver in deep dives. Usually these symptoms tend to appear below four atmospheres (98.4 feet or 30.2 meters). The condition poses no significant physiological or anatomical threat to the diver except that there may be faulty judgement and poor decisions that can lead to other risks. Treatment is by ascending to a shallower depth and the symptoms disappear immediately. If one observes one's buddy exhibiting any of these symptoms, one is to encourage them to ascend to a more shallow depth.

Decompression Sickness

If the above behavior develops during ascent, end the dive. If on the surface the behavior continues, then nitrogen narcosis can be excluded and one should consider decompression sickness or other medical or psychological problem. Decompression sickness is due to nitrogen gas bubbling out of the blood or tissues upon ascent from a deep dive. Symptoms of decompression sickness depend upon where there is formation of bubbles of nitrogen gas. Poor coordination and behavior changes could occur but the more common symptoms of decompression sickness are:

Joint pain
Numbness or altered sensation in the face, arms, or legs
Weakness or paralysis
Loss of vision or hearing
Abdominal pain
Unconsciousness

These symptoms may begin while ascending, during a safety stop, at the surface, on the boat or shore, or several hours after the dive. A diver should have a high level of suspicion for decompression sickness if any of the symptoms mentioned above are experienced after a deep dive. Medical attention and treatment for decompression sickness should be initiated immediately.

The Recreational Dive Planner is meant to be very conservative in its recommended No Decompression Limits. Its use assumes that the diver is spending the entire duration of the dive at the maximum depth. The dive computer measures real-time nitrogen saturation of the diver and will allow for significantly longer dive profiles. Divers should always stay within the No Decompression Limits of the tables or the computer. A slow ascent that is 30 feet per minute (9 meters per minute) or slower is recommended and will protect the diver from the bends in most instances. Finally, a safety stop at fifteen feet for three to five minutes is recommended for any dive below 40 feet (12.2 meters). It is also very important to ascend from the safety stop to the surface at a rate not to exceed one foot every two seconds. This portion of the ascent represents the most dangerous segment of the gas expansion curve and should be duly respected.

The diver who has a prolonged bottom time that reaches or exceeds the No Decompression Limits (NDL) should follow the recommendations of the Recreational Dive Planner. For a dive that exceeded the NDL by no more than five minutes, the diver should make a safety stop at fifteen feet (4.6 meters) for eight minutes. If the NDL is exceeded by more than five minutes, a fifteen-minute safety stop at fifteen feet (4.6 meters) is recommended. No diving for the next six hours is recommended.

The diver with any symptoms of decompression sickness should have hyperbaric treatment as soon as possible. Calling for emergency rescue personnel is mandatory as soon as the problem is suspected. The rescue personnel should be alerted to the likely diagnosis and requested to transport the victim to a facility with a hyperbaric chamber. If the rescue personnel conduct the rescue with a helicopter or air ambulance, they must maintain as low an altitude as possible to prevent the problem from getting worse.

Management on-site should include removing wet clothing and warming the victim. Lay the victim down and deliver oxygen by mask until emergency personnel arrive. Laying the victim on their left side has been advocated. The rationale for laying the victim on their side is to prevent aspiration if vomiting occurs. Laying the victim on the left side (right side up) is an attempt to prevent a bubble from crossing from the right heart chamber over to the left chamber of the heart and entering the general circulation. This will occur only if the individual has a septal defect in the heart (hole in the wall that separates the right from the left chamber). Monitoring the victim's vital signs and neurological status are important to determine whether CPR may be indicated in a victim who is deteriorating.

Barotrauma

Due to the changes in pressure while diving, a diver exposes those areas of the body with compressible compartments to barotrauma (pressure induced injury). These compressible compartments are those filled with compressible gas. These are the sinuses, the middle ear, and the lungs. The intestines are rarely involved with barotrauma because the intestinal wall and abdominal wall are so pliable. The most common problem encountered by divers is barotrauma to the ear and sinuses. These spaces are encased within a calcified wall that will not distend or contract to accommodate pressure-induced changes in the gas volume. Although usually not considered an emergency, this problem can become an emergency under certain circumstances.

Barotrauma of the ears can occur simultaneously with that of the sinuses since the same predisposing factors that lead to one can cause the other. Factors that predispose to difficulty in equalizing the ears and sinuses are upper respiratory infection, allergies, smoking, masses in the eustachian tube (polyps, tumors, abscesses, and hematomas), alcohol, rebound mucosal congestion after decongestants, hormonal changes, and poor clearing techniques.

If a diver begins to experience headache, mouth or tooth pain, or abdominal discomfort while ascending it may be due to expanding air in the sinuses, tooth implants, or intestine. The diver should stop ascending and wait for a time to see if the problem resolves. The diver may descend slightly to see if this alleviates the problem, then ascend slowly. Avoiding carbonated beverages before a dive may help prevent intestinal gas formation and discomfort upon ascent.

Ears and Sinuses

Barotrauma of the ears can be divided into outer ear, middle ear, and inner ear pathology. The outer ear is the canal outside the eardrum. The middle ear is the space inside the eardrum, and the inner ear is the spiral shell-like structure (cochlea) that contains the nerves for hearing (acoustic nerve). Problems can involve more than one compartment of the ear anatomy. The disorders of the ear can also be divided into descent and ascent barotrauma. The more serious of the two is a reverse squeeze during ascent. This occurs when the increasing volume of gas in the ear and/or sinuses cannot escape. The diver must either stay down to avoid injury and discomfort or ascend and possibly compound the problem. There is no magic solution to this problem. The best course of action is to patiently try all the methods of equalization until air or time limits prohibit further attempts, then ascend and immediately seek medical attention.

Never forcefully try to equalize the middle ear when descending. Ascend and attempt to equalize at a shallower depth with gentle pressure. Most of the time this will take care of the problem. Forceful attempts to equalize can cause serious injury to the mucosal lining of the eustachian tubes. A mucosal intussusception can be produced where the lining of the canal is forced with air pressure to telescope into itself. This will block the passage of air from the middle ear and can be complicated by bleeding and severe swelling of the tissues.

Inability to equalize the middle ear while persisting to go deeper can lead to injuries that may cause pain, hemorrhage, or perforation of the tympanic membrane (eardrum). Injuries to the inner ear can lead to tinnitus (ringing in the ear), deafness, severe vertigo, nausea and vomiting, and disorientation and ataxia (poor coordination). In either scenario, any of the above symptoms demand a dive termination and medical attention.

Barotrauma of the sinuses is heralded by discomfort of the face or headache. Pain in the eye, ears, or teeth may accompany the sinus pain. Nose bleeding during or after the dive would confirm a significant sinus squeeze. The diver should consider medical evaluation if the symptoms persist or worsen.

The most commonly practiced method to equalize is by pinching the nostrils and blowing while holding one's breath. Swallowing, yawning, lifting the soft palate, elevation of the pharynx with upward contraction of the tongue (Frenzel maneuver), forward and downward thrusting of the lower jaw, and wiggling the jaw side to side may also be used as techniques to open the eustachian tube and equalize the middle ear. If the ears or sinuses cannot be equalized, terminate the dive.

Chest Cavity

Pulmonary barotrauma is a pressure-induced lung injury. The mechanism of this injury makes it a phenomenon that almost always occurs upon ascent. Air that escapes the lung and enters the chest cavity outside the lung is called a pneumothorax. If air enters the cavity where the major blood vessels, the trachea, and the esophagus are located in the midline we call it mediastinal emphysema. If the air enters the cavity where the heart is located we call it precordial emphysema. If the air enters the blood stream we call the flowing bubbles of gas an air embolus.

Avoiding breath-holding during diving and ascents will markedly reduce the incidence of these conditions. Certain disease states of the lung can predispose a diver to develop these problems. These are asthma, pulmonary cysts, pulmonary fibrosis (scarring of the lung tissue), pulmonary blebs, pleural adhesions, sarcoidosis, pulmonary infections and tumors, chronic obstructive pulmonary disease, emphysema, and a history of prior pneumothorax.

Treatment of pulmonary barotrauma depends on the severity of the problem and the complicating circumstances. If a tension pneumothorax develops, aspiration of the trapped air is indicated as soon as possible (See section on Pneumothorax). If the victim maintains adequate respirations and circulation they are to be treated with oxygen. Closely monitor the victim's vital signs and neurological status, with rescue breathing or full CPR being administered if indicated. Laying the victim down and keeping them warm and dry without giving anything to eat or drink is recommended until medical personnel take over.

Lipoid Pneumonia

This condition is most commonly encountered when air compressors have oily contamination of the compressed air that is used to fill divers' air tanks. The vaporized oil is inhaled by the diver and causes an inflammation of the lung tissue. The reaction may produce progressive symptoms and cause significant respiratory failure. The reaction of the lung tissue could have long-term effects leading to pulmonary fibrosis (scarring of the lung tissue) and heart failure.

The diver may experience no symptoms if minimal contamination of the air is present or may begin to experience shortness of breath and coughing in heavy contamination. If a diver begins to experience respiratory problems during the dive or senses an oily taste to their air, they should cease diving immediately. Buddy breathing while ascending may be considered but in most circumstances all tanks may have been filled at the same facility and possess the same contamination.

Elimination of the continued exposure to the contaminated air is the diver's first priority. If symptoms of shortness of breath and/or coughing are present, the diver may benefit from oxygen therapy until taken to a medical facility for definitive evaluation and treatment. Chest x-rays may reveal a diffuse inflammation of the lung tissue that may be reversible with steroid treatment.

Carbon Monoxide Poisoning

Carbon monoxide poisoning of a diver occurs when the air intake of the air compressor is exposed to the fumes of the motor of the compressor, boat's engine, or vehicles nearby. Although the carbon monoxide is colorless, tasteless, and odorless, it is usually accompanied by other byproducts of fuel combustion that may give the diver a clue of the dangerous contamination that exists. Because of the oily byproducts of fossil fuel combustion, a concomitant lipoid pneumonia can also occur.

Low concentrations of carbon monoxide may cause little or no symptoms. There is a direct relationship between symptoms and the blood concentrations of carbon monoxide. Carbon monoxide forms a bond with the hemoglobin molecule that is 218 times stronger than the chemical bond between oxygen with hemoglobin. Because of this reason even low levels of carbon monoxide contamination in a diver's tank may become compounded during the dive.

The symptoms of carbon monoxide poisoning begin with a band-like frontal headache, shortness of breath on exertion, dizziness, weakness, nausea and vomiting, and dimness of vision. These symptoms can progress to loss of coordination, rapid heart rate and respirations, loss of consciousness, and coma. If the problem is not corrected death will follow. The victims are consistently noted to have cherry-red skin, nail beds, and mucous membranes.

Prevention of this condition is achieved by filling or renting tanks at reputable establishments that undergo quality inspections routinely. In remote areas with unknown standards the diver may elect to use carbon monoxide sensors that are commercially available. Smelling the air in the tank as part of the pre-dive routine may disclose evidence of air contaminated with fumes.

Treatment is directed at removing the victim from exposure to contaminated air. If symptoms are encountered, the dive must be terminated at the first signs of problems or suspicions of contamination. Buddy breathing during ascent may be of limited value since in most circumstances all tanks have been filled at the same establishment and suffer from the same contamination. Once at the surface, administering high concentrations of oxygen therapy is the best treatment until the victim can be taken to a hyperbaric facility for further treatment. CPR may be needed for advanced cases of poisoning.

Oxygen Toxicity

Oxygen at high concentrations is a toxic substance to all body tissues. Oxygen concentration and duration of exposure are the two most important variables that dictate the likelihood of injury to the diver. The central nervous system and lungs are the two body systems that are at highest probability of exhibiting symptoms during oxygen toxicity.

The two parameters that will increase the risk of toxicity to the diver due to the oxygen concentration are the absolute concentration of oxygen of the inhaled air and the depth of the dive that affect the partial pressure of oxygen. Regular air has 20.8% oxygen. As the diver goes deeper the partial pressure of the oxygen increases. At five atmospheres the effect on the body of regular air is the same as if breathing 100% oxygen at the surface. Below 130 feet (39.6 meters) the diver is exposing the body to the partial pressures of oxygen that exceed 100%. If the diver is using enriched air the percentage of oxygen in the air is increased and the partial pressure of oxygen is correspondingly increased at each depth of the dive.

There is wide variability for the onset of symptoms from individual to individual, and within the same individual during different dives. The diver's general state of health is an important predictor of problems. The diver's state of hydration, fatigue, illness, and physiological state may increase the probability of symptoms.

The pulmonary symptoms take longer to develop than neurological symptoms and begin at levels of oxygen that are safe for the brain. At high oxygen tensions the neurological symptoms are therefore the first to appear. The most common neurological symptoms are vomiting without nausea, sleepiness, restlessness or fear, tunnel vision, dimness or blurred vision, flashes of light, ringing in the ears, dizziness, lightheadedness, facial twitching, and generalized or focal seizures.

The pulmonary symptoms may be the first to manifest themselves at lower concentrations at times of prolonged exposure. The pulmonary problems arise from absorbing the oxygen within the lungs and collapse of the alveoli (minute air packets). There may also be damage to the lung lining and the microscopic blood vessels within the lung tissue. There may be fluid buildup and congestion of the lungs that may lead to breathing difficulty and possibly permanent scarring of the lungs. Symptoms may include an irritation of the lungs at times felt as a tickling in the chest cavity that may progress to pain or burning. Cough usually is mild and occasional at first, but then progresses to become severe and persistent. Shortness of breath is progressive.

Prevention is by adhering to shallow dive profiles. If using enriched air (air with higher than normal concentrations of oxygen), the diver must understand and adhere to dive profiles intended for the specific concentrations used. Switching to a lower oxygen concentration if multiple concentrations of enriched air are available is advised. If mild symptoms begin, ascending to a shallower depth will usually cause resolution of symptoms. For severe symptoms the rescuers are to ascend with the victim following described methods. If the victim has neurological signs but no pulmonary symptoms, basic first aid and life support are followed without oxygen. If the problems include or are limited to pulmonary problems, administer oxygen to the victim at the surface in addition to basic life support until medical assistance arrives.

Unconscious Diver

The most serious and time-sensitive event underwater is encountering an unconscious diver. Injuries and conditions that may lead to an unconscious state are many, some of which may have nothing to do with diving itself. Strokes, seizures, heart attacks, shock, syncope, and many other sudden onset conditions statistically occur to a percentage of the population on an ongoing basis. It is only reasonable to conclude that with the growing popularity of diving, the likelihood of these conditions occurring to a diver will also increase. The physical and psychological stress during diving may also increase the potential of these conditions to any individual at risk. Losing consciousness may also occur from diving-related conditions such as contaminated air, anaphylaxis (from a sting, bite, or chemical exposure), barotrauma, oxygen toxicity, shock, carotid sinus syndrome, hypothermia, and decompression sickness.

The very first priority is to get the diver out of the water as soon and as safely as possible. This will require a proper ascent rate to protect the rescuer and to limit further injury to the victim. The victim's BCD should be emptied and the ascent should be controlled with the rescuer's BCD. Dumping the victim's weight is seldom necessary and could lead to an uncontrolled ascent rate. If the rescuer's BCD does not have the capacity to bring about positive buoyancy then the rescuer can use the victim's BCD to supplement the lift of the rescuer's BCD. The rescuer may find it easier to bring the victim to the surface while holding them from behind (See Figure 21 for Ascent with unconscious diver victim). This may facilitate access to their regulator and BCD inflator hose. The rescuer may reach around the victim's head and hold the regulator in the victim's mouth with their right hand. With his or her left hand the rescuer may reach over the victim's shoulder to gain access to the victim's BCD inflator.

Maintaining an open and clean airway is the next priority. Even unconscious or comatose victims will attempt respirations. It is therefore my recommendation that the rescuer be sure the regulator is in the victim's mouth, and if not it should be placed in the mouth and purged. Should the unconscious diver attempt a breath, they will receive air and not more water. An unconscious diver with the regulator out of his or her mouth would be assumed to have inhaled water at some point. In order to allow some lung surface area for exchange of gases, the rescuer may squeeze the chest firmly once or twice after the regulator has been replaced to evacuate some water from the lungs. The normal recoil of the chest wall will then cause the diver to inhale air in exchange for the purged water from the lungs. During ascent, the victim's jaw should be extended to open the airway and allow for air to escape the lungs. Intermittently squeezing the chest firmly will ensure purging of expanding air in the lungs during ascent. The normal recoil of the chest wall will function as a bellos and bring about a shallow inhalation to the victim allowing for rudimentary rescue breathing.

If the ascent becomes uncontrolled for any reason that cannot be compensated for, the rescuer is to let go of the victim and ascend safely on his or her own. Once at the surface one may elect to dump the weights of the victim after inflating the BCD to maintain positive buoyancy. The rescuer may elect to keep their own weights at

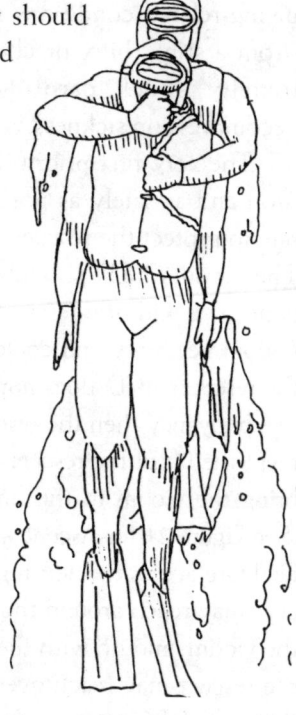

Figure 21 Ascent with unconscious diver.

the surface depending on the circumstances. The victim at the surface should be assessed for the need to initiate rescue breathing. Signaling the boat or shore for help and making an effort to recruit additional rescuers should be attempted while attending to the victim.

Entanglement and Entrapment

A diver may be restrained from continuing on with the dive for a variety of reasons. Getting tangled usually occurs with vegetation, nets, rope, and fishing line. Getting caught most frequently occurs during reef, cave, or wreck diving. Getting lost in a wreck or cave may be considered entrapment. A good buddy is one's best solution to resolving any of these problems. If entangled, one's buddy is in the best vantage point to assess and untangle the diver. Struggling, twisting, or spinning will undoubtedly make entanglement worse. The rescuer-buddy needs to be careful not to become entangled as well. The situation should be carefully assessed before the diver decides to either address the entanglement or go for help. If for some reason one's buddy is not there, removing the BCD vest may be the best option to untangle oneself. A sharp diver's tool may become an indispensable instrument to cut oneself free from vegetation or lines. The diver should always direct the force of the knife while cutting away from oneself or the entangled diver to avoid injury once the knife cuts through the line.

If caught in a reef or wreck, again, one's buddy is in the best position to help. If the diver tried swimming into too tight of an area, one's buddy could pull him or her straight back. If one swam into a wreck and was unable to find the exit, a buddy at the exit site could light the way out. If wedged into a tight corner, one's buddy may be able to supply the needed pull or push to get free. If unable to help, a buddy can go for help.

If the distressed diver's buddy is unable to make progress in a short time the situation should be quickly assessed to determine what may be needed to liberate the diver. The rescuer is to mark the site with a buoy if available, leave the primary air tank behind with the regulator, and surface with an emergency ascent bottle (Spare Air) for help. The buddy is to cautiously return with help, a buoy line to mark the area if not already done, equipment to free the diver, extra lamps, and another air tank with its own regulator. While on the surface, the rescuer should have the surface crew call for help, describe the problem in as much detail as possible to the surface crew, and direct the help to the area as soon as possible.

If one is hopelessly entangled or entrapped and there is no buddy available to help, air conservation and signaling for help are the only two options one has. Signaling should be done without expenditure of air. Do not use underwater air horns. Rapping on the tank should be done continuously as loudly as possible but without much movement to minimize fatigue and optimize air consumption. Signaling with one's lights should be used even during daylight hours and directed toward the entrance of the cavern, overhead, or wreck in order to gain the attention of a search party. Light batteries will last longer than one's air supply and battery conservation should not be a concern. If one has electronic communicators they should be used to call for help, stopping after each call to listen for any response or attempt by the rescue party to communicate.

Every diver may consider carrying a second bottle to increase the volume of air that is carried or in case of regulator malfunction. When cave or wreck diving, appropriate precautions and techniques should be followed as taught in specialty courses. A self-contained ascent bottle or a pony bottle will do for routine diving. The self-contained ascent bottle is smaller and can fit in a BCD pocket but offers only a few minutes of air. This, however, may be all you need to survive. A pony bottle, on the other hand, is larger and is another load to attach to an already heavy pack. The benefit of the pony bottle is that it will allow for more time.

Air is composed of 20.8% oxygen and the air that is exhaled still maintains a fairly high level of oxygen. This is why mouth to mouth resuscitation works to deliver sufficient oxygen to a victim. A diver who is trapped or entangled and needs to conserve air while a search is being conducted may use this concept to increase underwater airtime if in a very difficult situation.

The diver can inflate the BCD and breathe from the BCD, then exhale back into the BCD to reuse that air which will mix with the remaining air in the vest. This will decrease the oxygen concentration in the BCD air very little with each breath but the diver has not lost any air. As one breathes into the BCD the air will accumulate an increasing carbon dioxide level and a lowered oxygen concentration. The higher levels of carbon dioxide and the decreased oxygen will cause the diver to begin to experience air hunger and increase their respiratory rate. When the diver detects this tendency to increase the respiratory rate, it is time to change the air in the vest. At this point the air inhaled from the BCD can be exhaled into the water as usual. When the BCD is empty it can be refilled with fresh air from the tank. A diver's airtime can be significantly increased using this technique. This is also a good reason to keep the BCD washed and rinsed out.

Other potential sources of air in dire emergencies may include trapped air in wrecks, caves and cavern diving, and in overhead obstructions. This air is usually of poor quality but frequently contains enough oxygen to sustain life for a time.

Buddy Separation/ Lost Diver

Buddy Separation

Visibility and barriers will determine how or why there is a "separation." My definition of separation is simple: a visual or physical impediment to confirming your buddy is OK or being unable to give assistance. Therefore, if you can see your buddy but are unable to get to them to help, there is separation. Likewise, there is separation if you are five feet away from your buddy when there is two-foot visibility. All strategies for correcting buddy separation are aimed at confirming your buddy is OK, and if not, being able to give them assistance.

Separation prevention is the best strategy and should be a priority during all dives. **Never let your buddy out of sight!** If your buddy does get out of sight, getting back in sight is top priority. If you have communicators, talking to the other diver to let them know you don't have a visual fix on them until they are back in sight is mandatory. In excellent visibility a great distance between buddies can be tolerated comfortably. As the visibility decreases the proximity to your buddy should correspondingly increase. In very poor visibility a buddy line is recommended, or if no buddy line is available then handholding is the next best alternative. At times where there may be two or more factors affecting visibility such as fine bottom sediment with already murky water or during a night dive, a buddy line may be considered.

Visibility is one of the more important variables that can lead to buddy separation. Factors that can affect visibility are water movement, sunlight, bottom composition, suspended particulate material, outflow of nearby rivers or streams, blooming organisms, and the buoyancy control of the diver.

If the visibility is very good and one cannot find one's buddy, most of the time it is due to an unannounced ascent on their part. In excellent visibility, one should be able to identify a person on the surface and a quick survey of the surface may spot the missing diver. If the bottom is a distance downward then visual inspection of the bottom is swiftly completed. If one's buddy is not found, then a quick 360-degree scan is done twice (720-degree turn) to confirm your buddy is not nearby. Tapping on the tank with a tank-banger or one's dive-tool is begun to see if one gets a response. If there is a response then communication should continue until there is a reunion. Having a pre-planned audible code to signal one's buddy to ascend is helpful if buddies are unable to reunite. If no response is heard then a controlled ascent to the surface is recommended. If they are not there, a formal search is initiated.

In poor visibility, one can assume that one's buddy is usually not very far away when there is separation. If a diver goes a long time before checking on their buddy, then there may a greater distance between buddies in poor visibility and the likelihood of finding them without surfacing decreases. One can attempt to communicate with one's buddy by rapping on the tank and listening for a response. If a response is heard it is often difficult to discern direction due to the rapid speed of sound in water, but some idea of distance may be appreciated. If there is one-foot to five-foot visibility, swimming in a tight circle and expanding slowly is the best method to scan the surrounding area for one minute. If unable to find your buddy, then surface. If one can hear their buddy banging on their tank, one may continue to search for longer than one minute but not much longer than five. This is because there may be limited air on their part and they may be in distress, bringing a need for timeliness into the equation. It may be advantageous to surface and get more divers to help search for the source of the tank banging.

If there is a physical barrier such as a wreck, a coral formation, cave, cavern, or the like that your buddy has penetrated, and they are not visualized, do not enter immediately. Swim to the entrance of the barrier and inspect the other side or interior (whichever the case may be) to see if your buddy can be visualized. Begin by giving an audible signal and listening for a response. This is usually unnecessary if the buddy team is using communicators. If no response is heard, the specifics of the situation and the familiarity of the location will dictate whether one should enter and search, wait outside for several minutes to see if one's buddy exits, or make a controlled ascent and call for help. If one does find one's buddy and they are somehow entangled, tethered, or caught, and your assistance is either unsuccessful or you are unable to assist, a quick assessment of the problem must be completed in an expeditious manner to determine what may be needed to liberate the distressed diver. The rescuer may then consider removing their tank to leave it with the distressed diver and ascend with the self-contained ascent bottle if possible. The next priority would be to return as soon as possible with another tank (preferably with its own regulator) and any tools that may be helpful after activating the EMS system while on the surface.

Communicators do add a considerable degree of safety and are an immense aid to knowing your buddy is OK when there is a separation. A diver can be advised what their buddy is doing, what their situation is, or where they are located. Communicating the separation to the surface can also be done with the use of a surface monitor. If your buddy surfaced while you were searching for them below, this could also be communicated from the surface to the diver.

Lost Diver

It is not uncommon for a buddy team to go off on their own during a dive. The specifics of the dive will dictate what a reasonable period of time would be for all teams to have returned. If that period of time has elapsed or if one member of a buddy team has returned alone, a search is in order. When a diver is noticed to be missing, a full headcount may reveal that more than one diver is missing. Resources must be expeditiously allocated to cover all aspects of a search. Radio or telephone contact should be made with emergency personnel to immediately mobilize maximum resources. Simultaneously, the most experienced and best-qualified divers are to quickly but carefully don their gear and begin an underwater search in teams. The rescue divers should be equipped with lamps and marker buoys in addition to the essential diving gear.

A recall system is of utmost importance to call back rescuers if one team has found the missing diver or if the missing diver surfaces. Electronic communicators are the perfect recall system as well as coordination tools for a search, especially if a surface communicator is also available. Surface personnel may be divided into groups depending on the availability of individuals. Two or more individuals may be given binoculars and assigned to search the surface for bubbles, the missing diver, and any rescue diver that may surface. Someone else may need to maintain contact with the radio to direct emergency personnel. A designated individual may mark the area with a marker buoy where the diver was last seen and keep an eye for anchor drag, currents, etc. Factors such as currents, surge, visibility, and available air must be taken into account. A diver near the surface or mid-water may be carried along with currents much faster than someone at the bottom.

There are commercial Diver's Beacons available that may be considered in certain dive conditions. These beacons emit a traceable signal to help expedite a rescue and can be worn by each diver in the group. Night or evening dives, rough water, and strong currents may produce conditions that lead the Divemaster to consider using these Diver Beacons.

Search Patterns

The most reasonable initial search should be along the surface in all directions. Searching with a quality pair of binoculars greatly improves distant detail, and wearing sunglasses with polarized lenses is a major aid to the rescuers to filter out glare. Bubbles around the vessel are searched for but may be difficult to see in the distance, especially in wavy conditions. A systematic search of the water and horizon for marker buoys or divers at the surface may reveal a distant diver's head, arms waving, or a sausage buoy. At night the searchers should be keenly looking out for any evidence of flashlights and during the day any evidence of a mirror reflecting the sun's rays. These attempts by the missing diver at signaling the vessel or shore may be limited by the waves, and only split-second glimpses may be perceivable by the rescuers. All music, engines, and other noises should be eliminated to keep an ear open for whistles, air horns, or shouts from the missing diver.

Using search patterns will save time by searching an area in a coordinated and systematic fashion. The expanding square and the reciprocal U-pattern are simple and efficient methods of searching (See Figures 22 and 23 for Expanding Square and Reciprocal "U" Search Patterns). In good visibility, a group of divers can cover a large area in little time. Kick cycles are routinely used to gauge the size of the pattern covered. The reciprocal U-pattern is easiest if the diver searches in a straight trajectory a set number of kick cycles and then makes two right turns. The distance between the two turns at the ends of the distance searched will depend on the visibility. He or she then travels the same distance in the opposite direction and makes two left turns. They travel the same distance again and then make two right turns, and so on.

The expanding square is easiest if the diver travels a set distance, say five kick cycles. He or she makes a right (or left) turn then travels seven kick cycles, then another turn in the same direction. The diver continues to add two kick cycles or more depending on the visibility with each turn, always turning in the same direction.

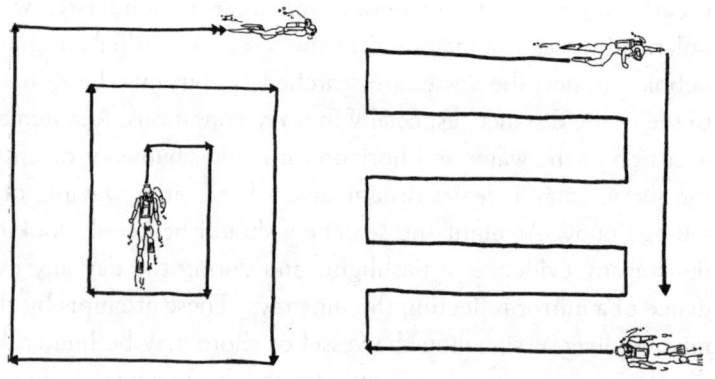

Figure 22 Expanding Square.   **Figure 23** Reciprocal "U".

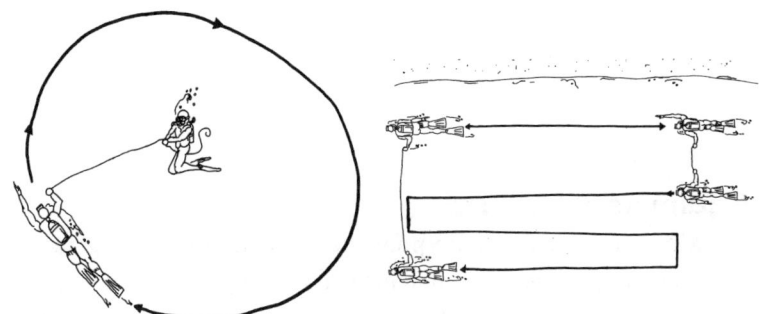

Figure 24 Expanding Circle.   **Figure 25** Shoreline.

In poor visibility, the expanding circle is the best option for searching (See Figure 24 for Expanding Circle Search Pattern). A central diver holds one end of a reel and lets out the line at a variable rate, depending on the visibility, to a second diver swimming in a circle. Obstacles will prevent this pattern of searching.

If along the shore or a wall, a diver can swim parallel to shore with a reel (See Figure 25 for Shoreline Search). The second diver swims parallel and at the same rate as the first diver with each trip back and forth. The diver closest to shore should swim back and forth along the same area to maintain a fixed reference point for the second diver. At each 180-degree turn the divers let out a length of the reel that would depend on the visibility in order to cover the area at increasing distances away from shore. This is similar to the reciprocal U but has a fixed reference point with a diver near shore to increase the accuracy of the search. The divers can signal when to turn with a series of tugs on the reel or with the use of electronic communicators.

Near coral or wrecks, divers must quickly and carefully inspect areas of potential entanglement or entrapment. The search should follow a logical pattern to cover the entire area. Rapping on one's tank near entrances of enclosed or overhead areas may elicit a response. A conscious diver who is in peril and alone should continuously rap on their tank or attempt to communicate electronically.

Equipment Failure

Most problems may be preventable with good diving technique and proper gear maintenance. There are occasional failures that may not be foreseen. The impact of any malfunction on any individual diver should not be underestimated. Stress and anxiety can compound even a minor problem with equipment and precipitate a panic state. A large number of problems are encountered due to misuse, not malfunction. As the reader will see, one's buddy is the single most important source of assistance during just about any type of equipment malfunction. This underscores the importance of always diving with a buddy and maintaining close proximity and vigilance over each other.

Tank

Fortunately, tanks are of a simple design and the valve almost never malfunctions. The "low-on-air" and "out-of-air" scenarios should be able to always be avoided with frequent checks of the diver's gauges and properly timed ascents. Vigilance to the tank pressure cannot be stressed enough. Tank size may be a factor in low air situations. A tank of proper size should be chosen for the size of the individual and the type of dive planned. Having a second tank is always a wise decision. Either a pony bottle or an emergency ascent bottle will ensure that even with an out-of-air scenario the diver will still carry enough air to reach the surface. These bottles may also be needed just to have enough time to gain the attention of one's buddy if out of air at depth.

Buddy breathing or the use of the alternate second stage of one's buddy is the best option when low on air or out of air.

It should be stressed that if one buddy is low on air it is likely that their buddy will also be low. The double consumption of air on one tank will certainly deplete the second diver's air source rapidly. A proper ascent should be made at once. At times, there may not be enough air to make a proper safety stop. The divers in this circumstance should attempt to stay down at fifteen feet (4.6 meters) to complete as much of the safety stop as possible. If the tank's air was consumed to near empty, it is likely that the depth and duration of the dive would certainly warrant this safety stop to prevent problems. The divers should utilize all the air within the tanks without concern about sucking the tanks dry and risking damage to the tank. The diver's health certainly is more important than the value of two tanks. Keeping a spare tank at a 15-foot safety bar or at 15 feet on the mooring or anchor line would obviously be the solution to this scenario.

BCD

Buoyancy emergencies due to improper use commonly arise when the BCD is used improperly to compensate for an overweighted diver and during panic situations. Leaks, inflator malfunction, and low or out of air circumstances may lead to BCD malfunctions. BCD leaks are best managed with the help of one's buddy. Using the BCD of one's buddy to make a controlled ascent for both divers can usually be managed. The buddies should hold each other and swim upward aggressively to help compensate for the extra weight of the second diver that the single BCD may not be able to lift. Dumping their weight is rarely necessary, although if dumping weight is required at depth it should be done in a step-wise fashion, unloading the smallest amount of weight at a time that will allow for an ascent with vigorous upward swimming on the part of both divers. As ascent is achieved, the difficulty to continue to ascend should diminish as their exposure suit expands.

BCD power inflator malfunctions may be due to a valve stuck in either the open or closed position. Valves stuck in the closed position are likely due to hardening of dirt within the valve. If the valve has dirt or contamination around the stem of the inflator button, it may lead to a variable amount of leakage due to the button becoming stuck in the down position and the diver will experience buoyancy difficulty due to continual inflation of the vest. If the button returns to the closed position but continues to inflate the BCD, one should suspect a damaged valve or valve seat. The diver should simply disconnect the quick-release and make oral adjustments to ascend and terminate the dive.

The oral inflator may malfunction due to a broken spring. The button usually moves back and forth easily if this is the case. If the button stays depressed it is usually due to dirt or contamination along the valve stem. Depressing the valve several times in rapid succession may resolve the problem, but the system should be cleaned and serviced anyway. If the valve improperly seats or is dirty it may cause leakage from the BCD. Depressing the button several times in rapid succession may temporarily resolve the difficulty.

If the valve is stuck in the closed position, oral adjustments are made as required to maintain buoyancy until the diver is at the surface. If the inflator valve is stuck in the open position and uncontrolled inflation of the BCD is occurring, the diver can easily disconnect the quick release valve of the hose to the BCD. An ascent should be able to be done normally since during ascent it would be required to empty the BCD as one ascends to maintain a proper ascent rate.

Tank slippage is not an uncommon problem, especially if the harness is dry when strapped to the tank. Wetting the straps before placing them on the tank then lifting the harness to check the hold is always advised. A double tank strap design on the vest will decrease the likelihood of this eventuality.

A good buddy will keep an eye on the other diver's gear and catch tank slippage early. If the tank slips all the way through the harness it may pull the regulator out of the mouth of the diver and lead to a panic. The tank will rarely fall far from the diver since the BCD hose should keep it in proximity. The best course of action is to have one's buddy correct the situation right then and there by pushing the tank back into the harness and strapping it in tightly. Obviously the priority is to give the diver an air source before adjusting the tank.

In an out-of-air situation the diver will need to buddy breath or use their buddy's alternate air source and orally inflate their own BCD to achieve neutral buoyancy. A diver should then purge the BCD as required upon ascent. Remember that the buddy's tank, which obviously will also be low on air, will deplete his or her air at twice the rate.

Weights

Weights do not malfunction. They add negative buoyancy to the diver to be able to descend at the beginning of the dive. The problems with weights are usually due to misuse, too much, or too little. Wearing the weight belt under the vest or exposure suit is an infrequent but potentially deadly practice. Having the weights slip off or dumping the weight is another source of potential disaster.

If a diver is over-weighted and unable to initiate an ascent or is descending uncontrollably, the diver may need to dump some weight. Having integrated weights or a pocketed weight belt makes dumping small increments of weight much easier. The smallest amount of weight is dumped that will stop the descent and allow initiating an ascent with vigorous upward swimming. Assistance from one's buddy and their BCD will reduce the amount of weight that will need to be dumped. If a conventional weight belt is used, always hold the end opposite of the belt buckle while removing the weight to prevent all of the weights from slipping off the belt.

If a diver loses all of their weight and is in an uncontrolled ascent, there are three main methods of slowing down. The first is with the help of one's buddy who can empty their BCD along with the BCD of the diver in distress and attempt to slow the ascent to a safe rate. If the divers continue to ascend at an unacceptable rate, the buddy should let go and slow their own ascent before two divers are at risk of injury. Getting to a mooring line or anchor line will also resolve the ascend problem. If in proximity to a mooring or anchor line, the diver should swim toward the line on a downward angle to reduce the rate of ascent while getting to the line (See Figure 26 for downward swimming to mooring line).

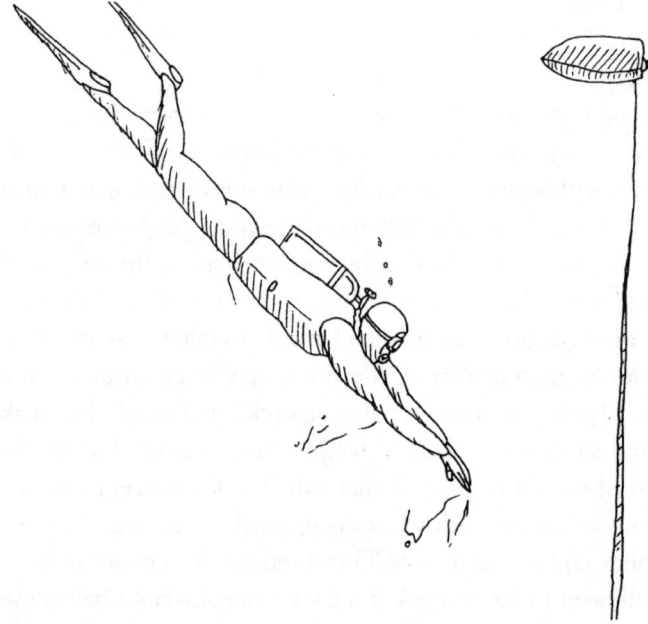

Figure 26 Swimming down and toward a mooring line during uncontrolled descent.

A "spread eagle" technique in a horizontal position such as sky divers use will increase the resistance to moving through the water and slow down the ascent (See Figure 27 for Spread Eagle Position). This technique has the disadvantage of not being able to further slow the diver if the ascent rate is still unacceptable. The "inverted" position where the diver is head-down and vigorously attempting to swim to the bottom is another method to slow down one's ascent (See Figure 28 for Inverted Ascent). This technique can be adjusted and fine-tuned to control one's ascent rate. If the downward swimming results in descent, the diver can slow down their swimming until the diver can confirm with their depth gauge that they are ascending. The pace at which they ascend can be adjusted to maintain a proper ascent rate until their feet reach the surface.

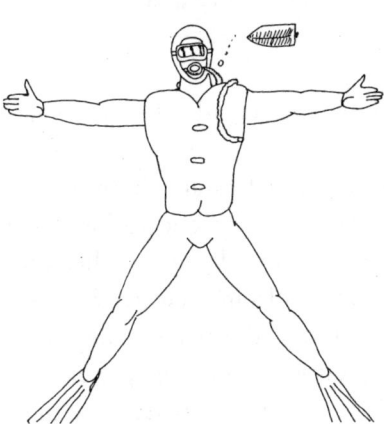

Figure 27 Spread-eagle position to slow down uncontrolled ascent.

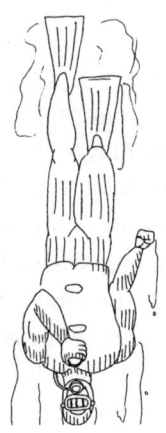

Figure 28 Inverted ascent position.

Regulator

Modern regulators are quite reliable but still require regular maintenance. Most regulators are manufactured so that in case of malfunction they become stuck in the free-flow position as opposed to the closed position. Divers should practice the technique of breathing with a regulator in free-flow for this eventuality.

Cold water diving may be a common cause for regulator freeze if the equipment is not intended for extreme temperature conditions. Using regulators with the proper parts and materials for extreme temperature diving is essential for safe cold water and ice diving.

The alternate second stage, the emergency ascent bottle, and one's buddy are the solutions to most regulator malfunctions. Familiarity with one's own equipment and that of one's buddy as well as techniques for buddy breathing are vital.

If the first stage malfunctions and there is air in the tank, one may get air directly from the tank valve using a free-flow technique. The valve may be turned off between breaths to conserve air. This technique is difficult and may result in tooth and mouth injuries, but in a bind it could be a diver's only source of air.

Fins

Fin problems are encountered in a remarkably high number of underwater emergencies. Many of the problems with fins are associated with other difficulties. Lost fins are the most common condition encountered. This may be due to having the wrong size or having the straps too loose. Panic or other stressful situations may also lead to fin loss from excessive leg movements. Fin loss may itself precipitate the panic state, lack of propulsion leading to buoyancy difficulty, or fatigue. Some documented cases of diver death have been in association with diving without fins. Fins are mandatory equipment for diving; they need to be the proper size and adjusted to the proper tightness to avoid difficulties.

If a diver looses a fin, efforts should be made to retrieve it. The best course of action would be to maintain neutral buoyancy and allow one's buddy to retrieve the lost article. If the fin cannot be retrieved, the disabled diver should ascend at an appropriate rate with their buddy and be towed to the boat or shore. The disabled diver may assist in the tow as much as possible with their single fin to prevent their buddy from becoming fatigued.

Mask

Problems commonly encountered with masks are due to fogging, leakage, and loss. Fogging is more of a nuisance than anything else. A clean lens that is treated with an anti-fog solution is optimal for clarity. Anti-fog solutions need to be used with caution since they can cause significant eye irritation if not rinsed out well, especially if contact lenses are being used. If fogging occurs, the diver may allow a small volume of water in the mask and use it to rinse the lens periodically. The diver simply looks down and moves the head in a circular motion to rinse the lens. Leave the water in the mask to rinse the lens again and avoid fogging the lens while purging the mask.

Leakage may be a problem with poor-fitting masks or those with a torn or broken skirt. Pre-dive assessment of the masks' condition and fit are very important. Masks with a purge valve leak much more often than those without. If the mask is not snug, air may leak out through the top of the mask and allow the valve to leak. Mucous or other debris may get caught within the purge valve and cause leakage as well. A dirty or old mask with a warped or defective valve is useless.

Loss of a mask may be due to strenuous activities, getting kicked, coming in contact with an underwater structure, colliding with another diver, or a panic state. Loss of the mask may easily precipitate a panic state on the part of a diver. Trying to maintain calm is the best course of action if one's mask is lost.

Initially closing one's eyes and pinching one's nostrils will help to regain one's composure. Once breathing has normalized, the diver may attempt to open their eyes to gain some visual cues about their surroundings. Holding the nostrils is not necessary, but some divers may find this more comfortable to ascend and finish the dive.

Seasoned divers who have a greater degree of comfort underwater will have a much easier time dealing without a mask than a novice diver. If the diver is overly anxious or in a panic the buddy may attempt to give them their mask to stabilize the situation, but be very careful not to loose both masks. If in doubt about handing over your mask, don't. Keep it and stay in control of the situation. One may have to deal with a diver in a state of panic until one reaches the surface.

Gauges

Gauge and computer malfunctions are not common with the more modern instruments. The most common malfunction of computers is a dead battery cell. Changing the battery every two years whether it's needed or not is wise. Many computers will allow for divers to change the battery themselves, while many models require sending the computer to the manufacturer to be serviced in order to change the battery. This may be one feature to look into when deciding which model to purchase. Should the computer malfunction, one's buddy is in the best position to offer assistance to surface at a safe rate.

Blowout of the high-pressure hose to one's gauges or of the gauge itself rarely causes injury underwater but may lead to a stressful or panic situation. It will also result in a rapid loss of tank pressure. The situation may be quickly controlled with the help of one's buddy. Take the alternate second stage of ones buddy to maintain a reliable air source. One's buddy should then shut off the tank valve to eliminate the free-flow of air under high pressure into the water. A proper ascent is then made together.

Marine Organism Attacks and Poisonings

Marine animal attacks are uncommon and deaths even more unusual. Still, care needs to be taken when exploring the aquatic environment. Danger may lurk in the least expected encounters. Fluffy, delicate, floating creatures could inflict deadly toxins and extremely painful stings as can colorful, delicate, small worms. That apparently slow and defenseless snail may possess the ability to deliver lethal poisons with lightning strikes. Bashful fish and snakes can attack with blinding speed and deliver mortal doses of venom. Known marine predators need to be respected and a diver's focused attention is warranted in their presence. Keeping one's hands to oneself may be a way of keeping one's hands.

The marine animals that are responsible for the majority of attacks are jellyfish, sea snakes, scorpionfish, stonefish, stingrays, cone shell, sharks, morays, and crocodiles/alligators. This list is comprised of organisms that are dangerous because they pose a threat in one of two ways: venom and/or attacks. Many attacks are in response to a perceived threat, while others are predatory behavioral instincts.

It is quite common to sustain an abrasion, puncture wound, or laceration while diving. These wounds quite commonly become infected and require special attention. All wounds need to be cleaned and antibiotic ointment applied until it is completely closed. Medical attention should be sought if a wound does not heal within two weeks. Many wounds need to be attended to immediately. Judgement and common sense will dictate which injuries are to be treated on one's own. If in doubt, always err on the safe side and seek a medical opinion.

Jellyfish and Coral

Jellyfish and coral are members of the same family and possess similar defense mechanisms. The most common stings are due to jellyfish such as the sea wasps and thimble jellyfish.

The more serious encounters occur with the Portuguese Man O' War (See Figure 29 for Portuguese Man of War), although in individuals who have a severe sensitivity to the jellyfish toxin much smaller species may pose a life-threatening risk. Death after becoming entangled in the stingers of jellyfish can come as soon as three minutes or can occur days later. The scars in survivors can be extensive. Rescuers attempting to help a victim of severe jellyfish stings must be extremely cautious not to become victims themselves. The microscopic toxin packets called nematocysts continue to be activated each time pressure is applied to the area involved. The rescuer must avoid rubbing on the affected area to prevent getting stung or discharging more nematocysts.

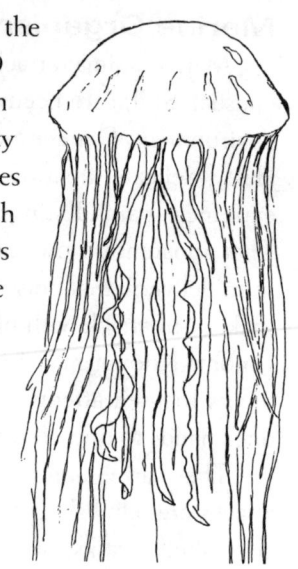

Figure 29 Portuguese Man O' War

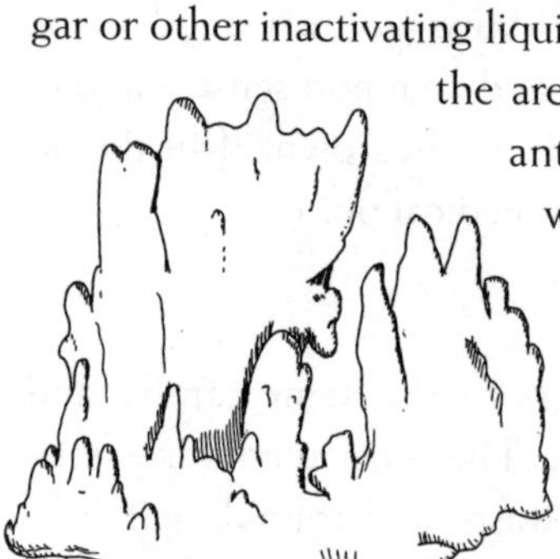

Applying vinegar or alcohol for 30 seconds will inactivate the undischarged nematocysts of jellyfish or coral. In case no alcohol or vinegar is available, the uric acid in urine may also inactivate the nematocysts. Although unpleasant, urine is usually sterile and poses no risk to the victim. Application of ice wraps after the vinegar or other inactivating liquid has been poured onto or soaked on the area will lessen the pain along with an anti-inflammatory medication. A firm wrap may reduce the absorption of the venom. Application of a steroid cream may markedly decrease the local inflammatory response.

Figure 30 Blade Fire Coral

Stinging coral (fire coral) is a relative of the jellyfish. Fire coral is usually a mustard color ranging from yellowish to olive with tan or brown tints. The tips are usually white with hairlike polyps. Poor buoyancy control or a strong current may cause a diver to rub up against these extremely painful organisms. (See Figure 30 for Blade Fire Coral) It is recommended that one use alcohol or vinegar to inactivate the nematocysts from coral. Do not rub the affected area upon the exposure until treated with vinegar or alcohol. Treatment with an analgesic and anti-inflammatory cream may also help.

Cone Shells

These docile-appearing large snails move deceptively slow (See Figure 31 for Cone Shell). They are armed with an organ that attacks with lightning speed and discharges a poison dart with extremely toxic chemicals. A victim will experience numbness and paralysis that begins in the area injured and spread to the rest of the body, eventually affecting the muscles of respiration. Treatment is aimed at preventing the circulation of the toxin and delivering CPR until an antitoxin is administered and medical support is given in a medical facility. Applying a broad tourniquet just proximal to the injury and applying ice to the area will reduce the circulation to and from the injury and reduce the spread of the toxin. This should be instituted as soon as possible at the time of the attack. If the victim experiences rapid progression of symptoms, the diver or buddy may use line or rope from a reel, a strap from a diver's tool sheath, or a watchband if need be. Immobilizing the extremity and application

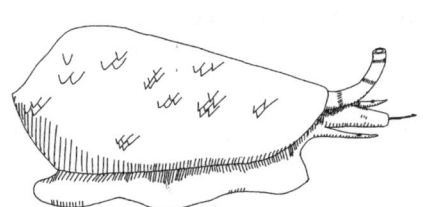

Figure 31 Cone Shell with dart protruded.

of ice will also reduce general absorption of the toxin. Calling for medical help is done immediately once on the surface and the victim is monitored very closely for paralysis and respiratory or cardiac problems. Rescue breathing is instituted if the victim stops breathing effectively (either fewer than 12 breaths per minute or moving too little air with each ventilation).

Stinging Sponges

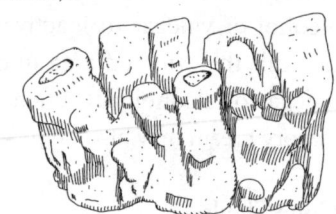

Figure 32 Stinging Sponge

Fire sponges are usually red, orange, or purple colored but may be any color, especially at depth where color has been filtered out. When touched with bare skin they will deliver a painful sting. They can produce itching, swelling, and extensive pain lasting up to a few days. The best rule is to look but not to touch anything. Application of vinegar followed by a steroid cream and oral analgesics are the preferred treatments.

Bristle Worms

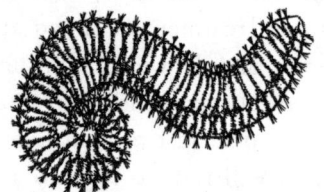

Figure 33 Bristle Worm

Bristle worms are brightly colored caterpillar-like worms that can grow up to about eight inches in length. They have a feathery appearance to them and can cause excruciating pain if touched by bare skin. The bristles detach easily and become embedded in the skin and cause pain for up to several days. It is recommended that the bristles be removed carefully with tweezers and a magnifying glass and the wound then cleansed with hot water. Application of alcohol, vinegar, or ammonia has also been advocated. Application of a steroid cream will help reduce the inflammatory response, pain, and itching.

Marine Snakes

Snakebites usually deliver a larger aliquot of venom than most other marine animals (See Figures 35 and 36 for Banded and Yellow-Bellied Sea Snakes). The volume of sea snake poison delivered is smaller than land snakes but is more potent and lethal. The initial treatment is immobilization and compression of the site to limit absorption of the venom. Application of ice will reduce absorption by constricting the blood vessels in the area. In severe circumstances a tourniquet may be considered. Careful monitoring of the victim's neurological and cardiovascular status is required until medical personnel take over. Most importantly are the victim's ability to maintain normal breathing, blood pressure, and heart rate. CPR may be needed. Use of anti-venom is advantageous but it is unlikely that a dive group will possess the appropriate anti-venom for these circumstances, given that the multiple species of venomous snakes may require different anti-venom.

Sharks

Most shark attacks are of swimmers at beaches or on the surface. Scuba divers have sustained relatively few attacks. Divers who have been attacked have some common characteristics. Victims are usually away from their buddy or group, engaged in spearfishing or feeding, or provoking the shark in some manner. Men are attacked overwhelmingly more often than women. Sharks are attracted to blood, bodily secretions, behavior suggestive of distress, and low frequency sound (See Figures 34 and 37 for Hammer-head and Reef Sharks).

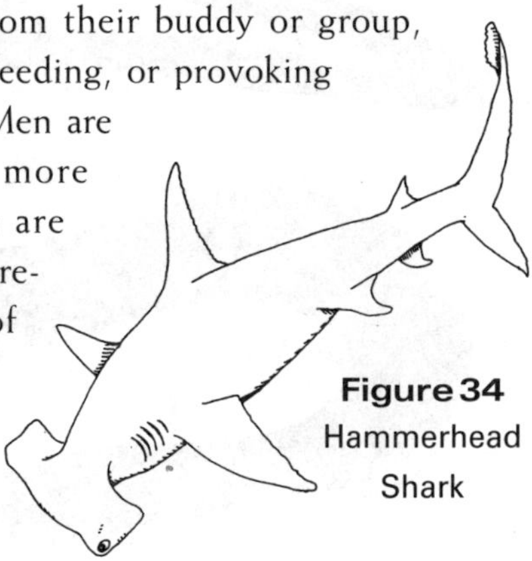

Figure 34
Hammerhead Shark

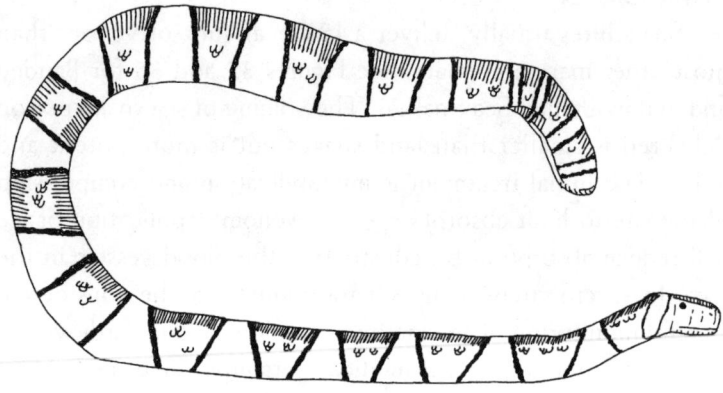

Figure 35 Banded Sea Snake

Figure 36 Yellow-Bellied Sea Snake

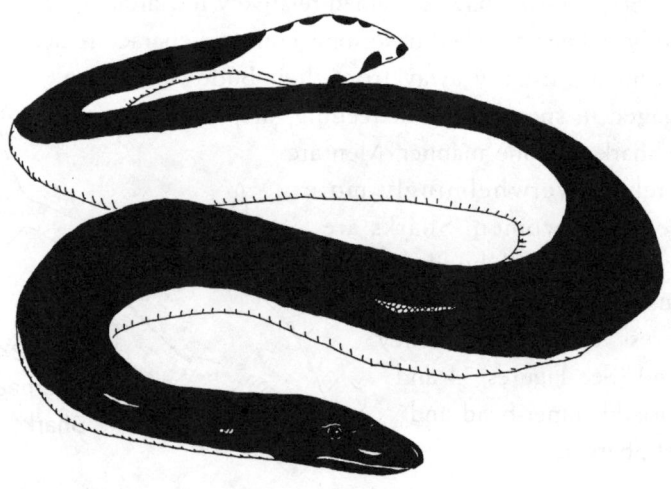

If a potentially aggressive shark seems to remain in the vicinity of a diver, the diver may elect to take cautious evasive action. Slowly swimming away

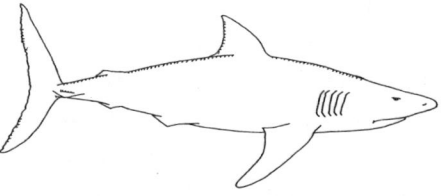

Figure 37 Reef Shark

while maintaining a vigilant eye on the animal is the best action. If near the bottom, the best strategy is to stay close to the bottom and swim as far away as possible before surfacing. If near the surface, swim away cautiously below the surface to not cause splashing at the surface which could attract predators. If there are formations or obstructions, try to get on the other side of these in order to escape outside the view of the animal.

A diver who is attacked should strike the shark or push it away in any way possible when the shark approaches. These efforts may prevent further approaches from the shark. If the diver has a speargun, it should be used as a shark billy and not fired at the shark. The diver's tool may be used as well. Stabbing the shark on the nose, gills, or eyes will be more effective to repel the shark than cutting it on the body. The shark's skin is very much like sandpaper. It is quite abrasive and can cause abrasions of exposed skin of the diver. Sharks have been reported to swim past a victim and sideswipe them with their bodies causing injury and bleeding. Nearby divers can do much to help repel further approaches by assisting in attacking the shark during its approach. Sharks almost never attack a group, even when there is blood in the water. It has been reported that sharks do not favor human meat. There are numerous reports that shark attacks on humans are limited to a single bite then the shark moves on. This has not been reported when there is a shark frenzy. During a feeding frenzy there may be multiple bites from multiple sharks in rapid succession.

Management of a shark attack is aimed at getting the injured diver out of the water as soon as possible and preventing other divers from becoming victims as well. Stopping blood loss may be done with direct pressure, packing of the wound, or a tourniquet, but it needs to be done immediately. The victims are to be carried out of the water with the head lower than the feet to maintain circulation to the brain in case of shock from blood loss. CPR may be needed as well. Oxygen therapy may be needed in case of aspiration of water, a rapid ascent, or a missed safety stop.

Crocodilians

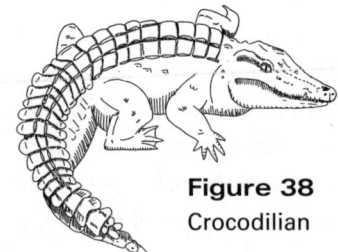

Figure 38 Crocodilian

Crocodilians include crocodiles, alligators, and caimans. These reptiles are especially dangerous organisms because they have the ability to attack on land and in water. They stalk their prey, hiding until they attack with veracious speed. Crocodilian attacks are rarely provoked. They are carnivorous creatures that seize any opportunity to feed (See Figure 38 for Crocodilian).

When an attack begins, the reptile takes hold of its prey with its powerful jaws and begins to roll in order to tear off large pieces of flesh that are swallowed quickly to follow with another bite. Crocodilians continue their attack until their prey has been devoured or they are killed. An attack by one crocodilian is frequently followed by other members that take advantage of the opportunity to benefit from the kill. They will pursue their wounded victim with the ability to follow their prey from water to land.

Attacks in water are difficult to guard against or defend against since this is their environment. The best advice is to avoid swimming or wading in waters inhabited by these predators.

Attacks on land may be avoided by not walking, picnicking, or camping along the banks or waterways inhabited by these reptiles. Being attentive to their hissing sounds may give a warning to the potential victim. Outrunning crocodiles is not likely as they are fast runners in short sprints. One may attempt to climb a tree, although crocodilians have been known to jump and stand on their hind legs to reach a victim. One may attempt to discourage their attack by throwing objects at them. If attacked, one should try to quickly injure them in the eyes. This may abort the attack. Prying open their powerful jaws is just about impossible and not an option.

Friends may try to help the victim by striking the attacking reptile in the eyes with sticks. Care must be taken that the attacking crocodilian or other reptiles in the vicinity do not attack a second person. If the attack is thwarted, the victim and the rescuers should evacuate the area immediately. Attention to the injuries should be cared for in a safe environment.

Moray Eels

There are many species of morays that inhabit the oceans. Although they appear quite sinister, they are not aggressive toward humans. They tend to shy away unless cornered and provoked. Most moray bites occur when divers are feeding them and the moray inadvertently bites more than the bait. The moray's teeth are thin, long, and very sharp and can inflict a deep wound. Their teeth are also teeming with microorganisms that will cause a significant infection if the wound is not attended to immediately. Cleansing the wound with an antiseptic, applying a sterile dressing, and getting medical attention is recommended.

The moray usually emerges from its hiding place at night to feed. During the day it will only dart out to bite the bait of diver's and return into its hiding area. The moray may bite a diver's finger that is feeding it. Rather than letting go of its food it will begin to twirl, tearing off the diver's digit. Should this occur, the diver is to apply firm pressure on the stump of the amputated finger to stop bleeding and seek medical attention immediately.

Barracuda

There are many species of barracuda but the great barracuda is the most commonly known to inflict attacks on humans. Barracudas are known to rely on their vision to hunt, and this is why attacks are thought to be caused by murky water and shiny objects worn by divers or snorkelers that may resemble their natural prey.

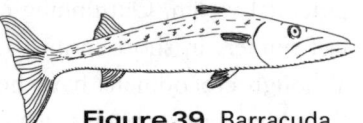

Figure 39 Barracuda

The attack of a barracuda is intended to slice its prey and make several passes to eat the pieces. Wounds are usually superficial but may bleed considerably and become infected. Pressure, cleansing with a disinfectant, and treatment with an antibiotic may be indicated.

Sea Urchins and Other Spiny Fish

The sea urchin does not attack but is found along shallow areas near beaches and entrance sites where divers enter and exit the sea. Stepping or falling on the long spines may inflict a painful and serious injury that at times may be poisonous with some species (See Figure 40 for Sea Urchin). Deep injuries to the face, chest, or abdomen can occur from spines that can reach over one foot long. The rescuer should attempt to remove the spines, being careful not to break them as they are being pulled straight out. These spines can become embedded and require surgical extraction in a hospital setting. Prolonged antibiotics may be required.

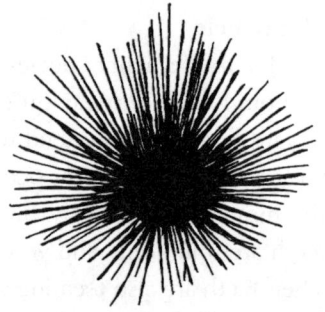

Figure 40 Sea Urchin

Injury with the venomous spines of rockfish and scorpionfish may be treated as would other venomous attacks with pressure, ice, immobilization, and possibly a tourniquet (See Figure 41 for Rockfish). Application of heat is beneficial to inactivate the venom and reduce the pain in the majority of situations. Stingrays and other spiny fish require prompt removal of the spines and cleansing of the wound. Hot water is good to bathe the affected area. Application of an antibiotic ointment until medical attention is sought would help prevent infection.

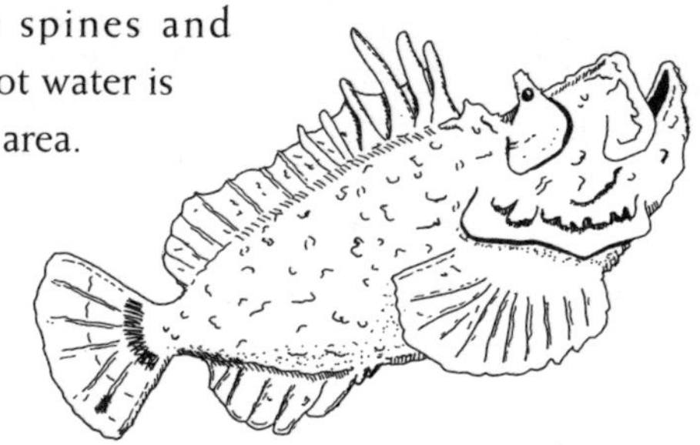

Figure 41 Rock Fish.

NOTES

CHAPTER FIVE

Surface Emergencies

Signs of Trouble

Emergencies on the surface may have begun underwater and the care of the victim must be continued on the surface. Other circumstances involving a distressed diver may be first identified on the surface. From below the surface, the signs of trouble of a diver near to or at the surface may include rapid ascent or descent rates, excessive movements of the hands and legs, dropping or loosing control of their gear, and lack of movement or no response to an attempted communication. The most obvious sign of a diver in trouble as seen from a boat or shore is a signal for help. This may be done by waving hands, blowing the whistle or horn, waving the sausage buoy, firing off a flare, or splashing the water around them. A diver in peril may not be signaling, but may be trying to cope with the problem at hand and proper interpretation of their behavior is important. Signs of trouble as seen from the surface are losing the mask, a mask on the forehead, splashing or thrashing about, bobbing over and under the surface of the water, and waving or splashing the water with the hand on the surface with the head underwater. Other manifestations of trouble may be throwing up, coughing or choking, screaming or yelling, lunging at or climbing on top of another diver, failure to gain their attention, an isolated diver at a distance from the rest of the group, and lack of movement of a diver on the surface. Recognition of a diver in trouble is key to initiating a rescue as soon as possible.

Dive Entrance

A significant number of injuries occur during entrances. Most injuries during shore diving are due to water movement (surges, waves, currents, etc.) and spiny marine creatures. Injuries on a boat dive may be due to entering onto a diver already in the water, striking the boat upon entry, or injury from a rocking boat once in the water. The most common equipment difficulties a diver has upon entering are problems with closed tank valves, adjusting to water temperature, lost mask or regulator, forgetting to put on the weight belt, and lack of buoyancy from an empty BCD or too much weight.

Entrance sites from shore need to be inspected for the pattern of water flow both near the shoreline and at a distance from shore. Knowledge of the tidal cycles in the area is wise and planning the dive just before low tide or preferably just before high tide will give the diver the slowest movement of water for the longest period of time. Shallows and reefs near shore can produce riptides that can move water seaward with incredible speeds and power. They can be recognized by an agitated and at times whitewater surface. Rapid seaward undercurrents at times cannot be appreciated from the turbulent surface. Strong shorebound surges can occur from funneling of waves between sandbars or large obstructions. Upwellings, on the other hand, can produce a gentle outward current on the surface to help the diver swim out from shore to the dive destination. Visibility may be improved by upwellings as well. In wavy water conditions it is best to find an open area with few or no formations or boulders. Knowledge of the coral reefs and barrier reefs in the area may be obtained from local Divemasters. Openings of the barrier reefs may be small and tricky areas to navigate on one's own, especially at night.

Divers, guides, and surface personnel need to vigilantly monitor the divers and their buddy's entrance, whether from shore or from a vessel. Any sign of distress is to prompt immediate assistance. Upon entry divers may give the "all OK" sign immediately upon entering the water as a habit without first checking their buoyancy or gear. Don't be fooled by this reflex response; keep an eye on the divers and one's buddy until they descend. Injuries may occur even if everything is OK because the divers are too close to the boat's hull before they descend. If a diver is injured or in distress, a crew member or Divemaster should be in a position to give immediate assistance. Tossing the distressed diver a flotation device with a line or entering the water and rescuing the victim may be required.

Boat Injuries

Divers at the surface are at risk of injury from the dive boat itself or from other vessels in the vicinity. Use of properly displayed dive flags and a current line will help reduce the likelihood of injury, although it will not eliminate these risks altogether. Following safe protocols for entering and exiting will further reduce the risk of injury from the dive boat.

Dive flags are intended to alert other boaters that divers are in the water. Unfortunately, there are boaters who are distracted, intoxicated, or just are not aware of the rules governing the diameter of the safe zone around a vessel engaged in diving operations.

The captain of the dive boat, the Divemaster, or a designated lookout should maintain vigilance in the area for bypassing vessels. If a vessel is approaching the dive boat needs to sound its horn or contact the vessel by radio and alert them to the divers in the vicinity. If contact with the other vessel is not successful, a visual signal may be given (i.e., arm waving, flood lamp, etc.).

The diver should also stay alert for the sound of bypassing vessels. Although direction may be impossible to discern, the crescendo (rising) volume of the engines will alert the diver that the boat is approaching. Sailboats may be of specific concern because their approach is silent and their keel usually extends deeper into the water than a powerboat of the same size.

A diver who hears an approaching powerboat should immediately descend to at least twenty feet (6 meters) in depth. Very large vessels may have a draft that is below twenty feet (6 meters) but they are most likely to heed dive flag warnings and remain a safe distance away. The diver may elect to stay at that depth until the sound of the powerboat begins to fade, or the dive boat sounds the call-back signal. The diver should look up and may circle slowly while watching the surface for the intruding vessel. Divers may elect to stay down for a short period of time to be sure that a second vessel may not be following the first.

The diver ought to be careful with any lines that may be in the area, either attached to themselves or that they are using to hold on to such as a buoy. These lines could become entangled or caught by the boat and the diver could sustain severe injuries from the sudden acceleration. Divers need to communicate their intentions and concerns to their buddy and take the necessary action to be sure their buddy descends and is free of lines as well.

Bypassing powerboats may injure the diver in one of two ways, either a blunt injury from the hull or a propeller injury. Depending on the position of the diver at the time of the impact, he or she may sustain injuries to any part of the body.

The blunt impact by the hull is likely to cause fractures and severe internal damage. Divers are likely to suffer from aspiration in addition to the injury from the impact. Propellers usually cause injuries that are parallel lacerations covering one side of the affected area. The depth of these lacerations may depend on the size of the propeller blades, which in turn is dictated by the size of the vessel. Amputations are not uncommon. Severe blood loss in a very short time span is the rule. Management will depend on the specific injuries incurred. Taking note of the offending vessel's name and description will be important for reporting the injury to the authorities. Many times the offending boater is unaware of the injured diver and continues to cruise away.

Injury from the dive boat may occur from a variety of circumstances. A diver ascending should always look up and extend one hand above their head to avoid hitting their head on the hull of the dive boat. When several divers are at the surface and ready to descend or exit, a current line will allow the divers to hold onto something other than the boat. A rocking boat is a danger to divers in the water. The hull, swim platform, propeller, or the ladder can cause severe head, neck, and bodily injury. A diver who is climbing out of the water could slip and fall onto a diver behind him or her. Equipment that is being handed up to the boat crew (i.e., underwater vehicle, lamps, cameras, weight belts, or tanks) may slip and fall onto a diver in the area. Even on a calm day when the dive boat is not rocking, a distant vessel may generate a sizable wave that can take the boat crew and the divers by surprise.

During the time that divers are in the water, the engines of the dive boat should be turned off. Divers most commonly exit the water from the stern of the boat in close proximity to the propellers. There is often a group of passengers and crew that are busy moving gear or situating themselves on deck of a rocking boat during the entrance and exit. An inadvertent push on the gear stick by a passenger or piece of equipment may throw the vessel into forward or reverse, leading to a disaster.

Lost at Sea

A diver or divers that have been carried away by a current or left behind when the dive boat leaves is a rare occurrence. This scenario can end in tragedy but foresight and the proper equipment may improve the likelihood of being rescued. The most immediate condition that can affect the diver is exposure and hypothermia. Dumping one's weights and floating horizontally on the surface may allow for reduction of heat loss by staying in the warmest water (surface water) and benefiting from the suns ray's to warm the exposure suit. Prevention of water flow through the suit will help reduce the heat loss. Swimming as little as possible does this. The swimmer may also reduce heat loss by getting into the tucked position to reduce exposed surface area (See Figure 42 for Tucked Position). Keeping the extremities tucked and flexed against the body will avoid water flow to the underarms, groin, and belly areas. The diver should keep their mask, gloves, and hood on to increase insulation. If there is more than one diver present, huddling close together may help conserve body heat (See Figure 43 for Huddling).

Swimming may be indicated if the diver is being carried by a current moving parallel to shore. The diver may elect to swim toward shore at a moderate pace to limit fatigue. If the diver is off shore to an island and the current has the potential of carrying the diver beyond the island toward the open sea, the diver may attempt to swim at a 45-degree angle against the current toward shore (See Figure 44 for Swimming Toward Shore Against Current). This will give the diver a better chance of approaching the shoreline before the current carries them past the island. If the current does carry the diver past the island, the diver may still elect to continue swimming the same course. The diver may be able to swim into waters that are protected from the current by the island (See Figure 45 for Swimming to Shore Behind Island). Once in still waters the diver may have a chance to swim back to shore on the other side of the island.

SURFACE EMERGENCIES

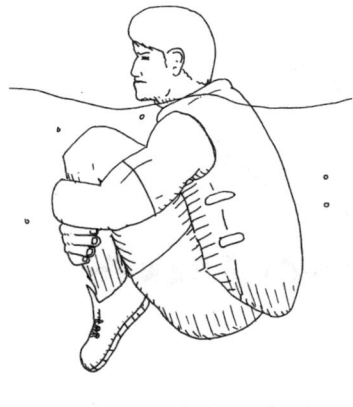 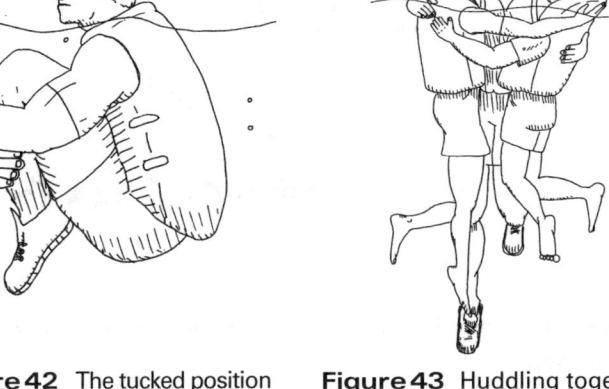

Figure 42 The tucked position will help conserve body heat during prolonged water exposure.

Figure 43 Huddling together to decrease heat loss.

Every diver should carry a whistle, an air horn, a light, and a sausage buoy on every open-water dive. A small mirror may also be of benefit for signaling. The light should have fresh batteries and a lanyard, and the sausage buoy should be clipped to the vest's shoulder D-ring to be sure it doesn't get away from the diver. The light should be saved for when it gets dark and a search is being conducted at night. A mirror can be used during daylight hours to help signal nearby vessels and planes but would be useless at night. The air horn can be heard at quite a distance, especially in calm water, but a whistle may be needed in an out-of-air scenario.

Signaling a vessel or search plane during the day is best done with the sausage buoy or mirror. Waving the buoy with a wide span is the best method. Holding the buoy as high out of the water as possible will improve the ability of someone on a vessel to see the signal especially in high waves (See Figure 46 for Waving buoy at boat). The use of the air horn can enhance the likelihood of being noticed by a passing vessel but will usually be worthless to signal a search plane.

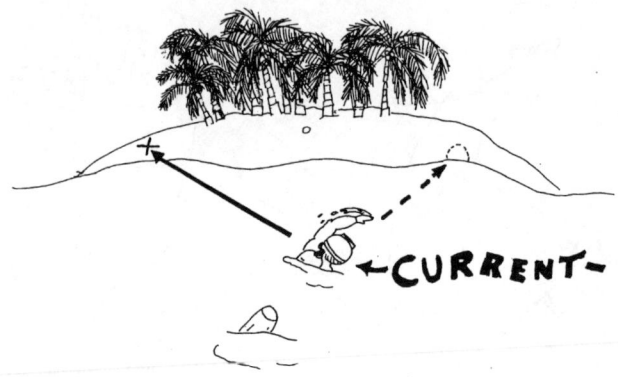

Figure 44 Swimming in a 45 degree angle against the current toward shore.

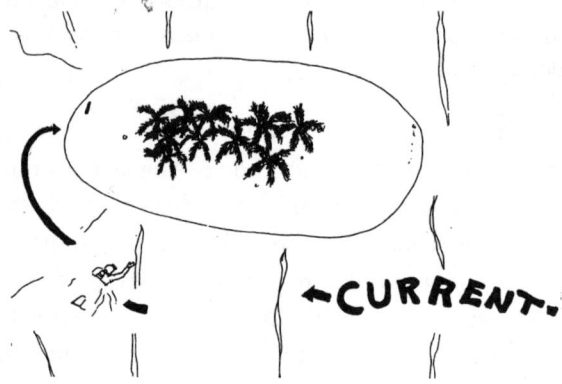

Figure 45 If the current carries the diver past the island, continuing on the same 45 degree coarse may carry the diver into waters protected from the current by the island and allow the diver to reach shore.

At night the lost diver will need to use the light to signal a vessel or plane. A bright light will be very noticeable in open water. Shining the light directly at the vessel or plane is the best method to signal for help. Signaling an SOS (dot, dot, dot, dash, dash, dash, dot, dot, dot) will immediately allow any party that sees the signal that it is a distress call and not just a curiosity.

SURFACE EMERGENCIES

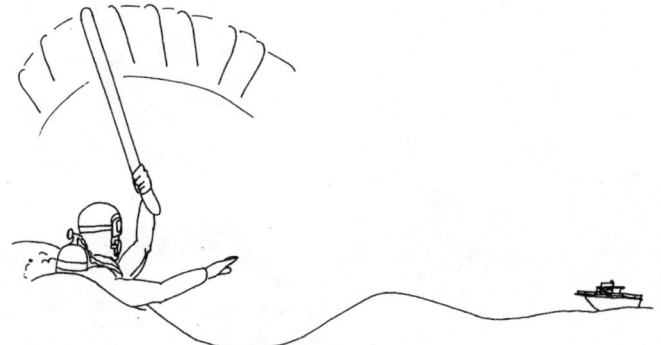

Figure 46 Waving the sausage buoy as high out of the water as possible to signal the boat for assistance.

During conditions of high waves where the lost diver is unable to shine the light directly at the vessel the diver may attempt shining the light directly at the vessel, as he or she comes over the peak of a wave and the vessel is in direct vision (See Figure 47 for Shining light at boat at peak of wave). When the lost diver sinks down to the trough of the wave they may shine the light at the sausage buoy to make it visible as the sausage buoy is waved as high out of the water as possible (See Figure 48 for Shining light at buoy at trough of wave). Use of the air horn and whistle will again enhance the signal of the lost diver.

There are commercially available diver's flares that can be used in this eventuality. The lost diver should consider waiting until there is an opportunity to use them when a vessel or plane will have the likelihood of noticing the flare. These flares last for several minutes and are quite bright, but if used at the wrong time will not be effective.

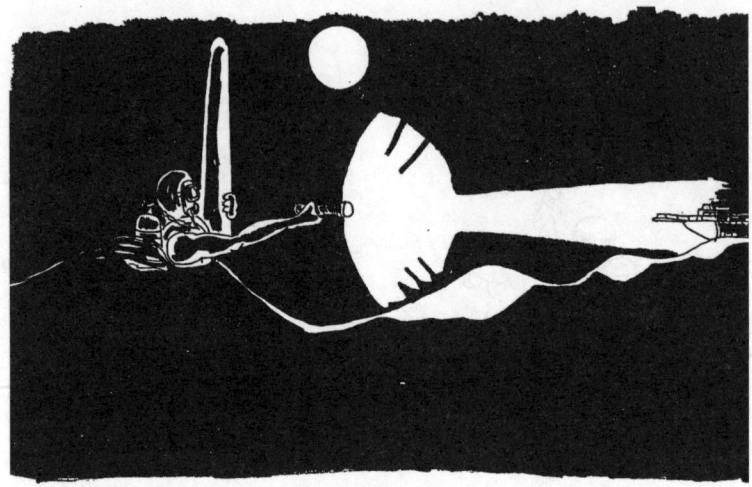

Figure 47 When at the peak of the wave a diver shines light directly at the boat.

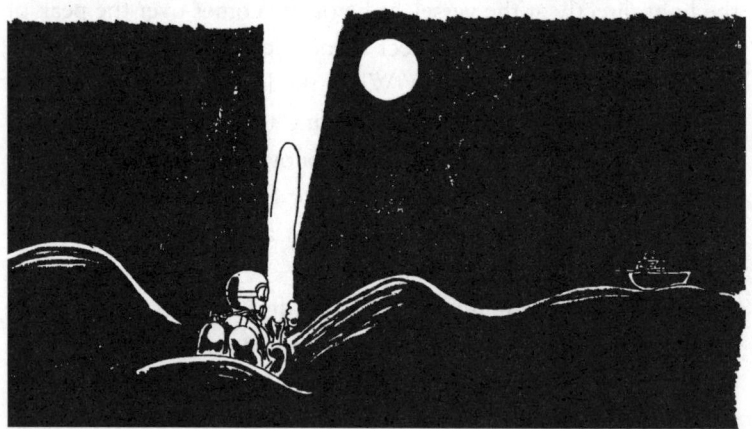

Figure 48 When at the trough of the wave the diver shines the light on the sausage buoy.

Fatigue

Due to the nature of boating and the equipment required for diving, divers may begin to feel exhausted even before donning their exposure suits. Heat, humidity, a rocking vessel, and an extended cruise to the dive site may all contribute to diver fatigue before the dive has begun. Carrying dive gear to the shore from the car, an extended surface swim to the dive site, and fighting current or surge may be contributing factors from a shore dive. Equipment difficulties may add a significant amount of energy expenditure to divers as well. The point is that a diver may suffer from fatigue even before descending. If this is the case the diver may elect to rest for a period of time at the surface before descending or cancel the dive to prevent exacerbating the condition during the course of the dive.

Fatigue may occur during the dive or toward the end of the dive. Most divers have time to rest during the safety stop at the mooring or anchor line at the end of the dive before attempting to exit and removing their gear. The swim to the boat is usually a short one from the line but the swim back to shore may be lengthy. Pacing oneself and changing the style of swimming (i.e., swimming on one's back) may help. Stopping to rest after notifying one's buddy is certainly acceptable.

The tired diver may be recognized because of falling behind the rest of the group, hyperventilating, slow and labored swimming, and by them communicating their condition to you. The rescuer is to help them establish positive buoyancy by assisting them in inflating their BCD. Care must be taken not to inflate the BCD to the point that the victim is unable to inhale from the pressure of the vest. Keeping their regulator in their mouth makes breathing much easier. If they are low on air, then their snorkel or the rescuer's octopus may be used. Resting is recommended before resuming a slower and more leisurely swim or tow to the shore or boat. The rescuer may elect to use any of the described towing methods depending on the condition of the tired diver (See Figures 49 to 51 on page 157 for towing methods.)

Panic

The diver in panic at the surface may manifest the same behaviors as may be seen in a panic diver underwater. The rescuer should approach a panic diver with caution. Approaching the distressed diver on the surface with a flotation device extended in front of the rescuer will give the panic diver something to grasp. This will assist them in buoyancy and protect the rescuer from being overcome from the panic diver climbing over them. The rescuer may get control of the panic diver only by getting behind them and holding them by the tank, tank valve, or the BCD harness. Getting behind the panic diver may be done by swimming around them while maintaining a safe distance or by descending under the panic diver and surfacing behind them.

Obtaining a hold of the diver's BCD from behind is the recommended approach to avoid injury from the panic diver's uncontrolled behavior. Inflating their BCD by reaching over the panic diver's left shoulder to gain access to their BCD inflator to establish positive buoyancy is the first priority. Dropping their weight belt may be considered but is not usually needed. Towing them back to shore or the boat using the tank-straddle tow technique is the next priority (See Figure 49 for Tank Straddle Tow). The rescuer may try to calm them down but these attempts may not be effective. Getting the diver to a line, boat, or other object to hold onto may at times help abort the panic attack.

If a diver in panic does get a hold and begins to climb over you, quickly get hold of your mask and regulator to avoid losing them. The last thing a panic victim will want is to go under. A rescuer can use this to their advantage by intentionally descending immediately upon the assault. The diver in panic will instinctively release them in an attempt to stay at the surface. The rescuer may need to take precautions from being kicked on the way down and evaluate whether it would be worth while attempting to get control of the panic victim from behind or to keep one's distance while continuing to monitor the situation. A small rescuer attempting to get control of a large panic victim from behind may become overpowered and injured. This approach may not be worth the risk. Careful monitoring of the panic victim and signaling for help (recruiting additional rescuers or obtaining a flotation device) may be the wisest form of management.

Towing

Upon occasion circumstances will arise that will require one diver to tow another diver from one point to another. There are several methods of towing a diver, each with its advantages and disadvantages depending on the particulars of the victim. All diver tows are done with inflation of the victim's and the rescuer's BCD. Inflation of a sausage buoy may help alert the boat or shore of a problem. Sounding an audible signal may assist in getting the attention of shore or boat personnel. Acquiring any flotation device will help the tow process. Dropping the weight of the victim may be considered, as it will give them better buoyancy and less drag. Multiple rescuers make for a quicker tow, better monitoring of the victim, and decreased fatigue. Panic diver tows are best conducted from behind the diver by holding both sides of the vest to prevent the victim from turning around. Holding the victim's tank between the rescuer's knees (straddle-tank tow) has been advocated to further prevent the panic diver from turning around and overcoming the rescuer, although this will markedly slow down the rate of tow (See Figure 49 for Tank Straddle Tow).

The rescuer has the disadvantage of not being able to see where they are going during the tow due to swimming backward. Should the panic diver get free of the rescuer, control from behind may be reestablished by descending and resurfacing behind the victim.

The underarm tow (Do-Si-Do tow) where the rescuer is beside the victim is beneficial to keep a closer eye on the condition of the rescued diver (See Figure 50 for Do-Si-Do Tow). The rescuer places their arm under the underarm of the victim and around behind the victim's head. This tow is required if mouth to mouth resuscitation is being given during the tow. It is a somewhat slow and cumbersome tow for the rescuer on long distances but allows for the best observation of the victim.

The tank-valve tow is conducted from behind the victim (See Figure 51 for Tank Valve Tow). The rescuer holds onto the victim's tank valve and the rescuer swims on their side toward their exit destination. This tow offers slightly more freedom for the rescuer and achieves a slightly faster pace as well as allowing the rescuer to see where they are going. This tow also allows the victim to assist in the tow by swimming while on their back, which further increases the pace of the tow and decreases the rescuer's rate of fatigue. The rescuer has less ability to monitor the status of the victim during this tow and may need to stop to check on them if needed.

The foot-shoulder push is more comfortable for the rescuer for long-distance towing (See Figure 52 for Foot-Shoulder Tow). It allows the rescuer to simultaneously keep an eye on the victim and to see where they are going as the tow is being performed. The rescuer should maintain a steady and paced kick cycle, otherwise he or she will fatigue and be of less help to the victim and themselves. The victim will be unable to assist in the tow with this method.

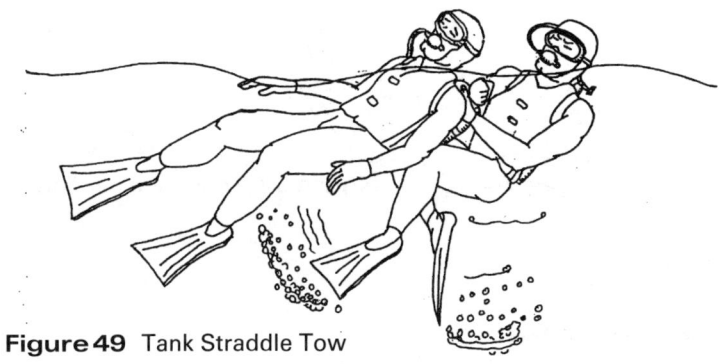
Figure 49 Tank Straddle Tow

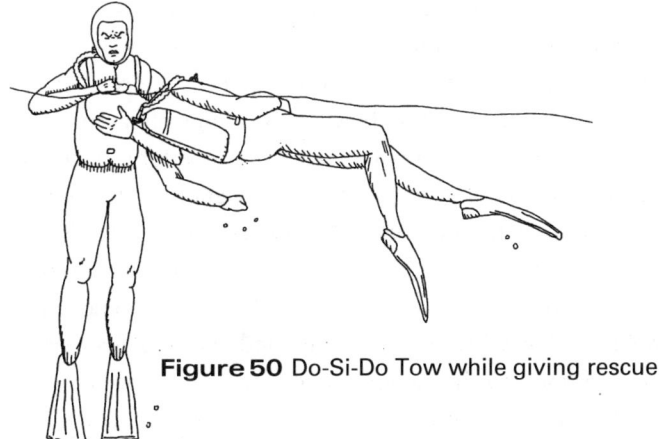
Figure 50 Do-Si-Do Tow while giving rescue

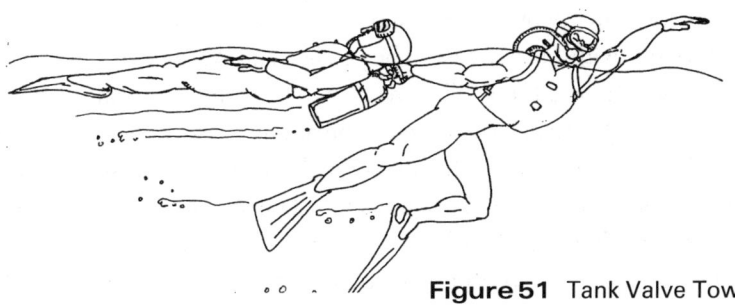
Figure 51 Tank Valve Tow

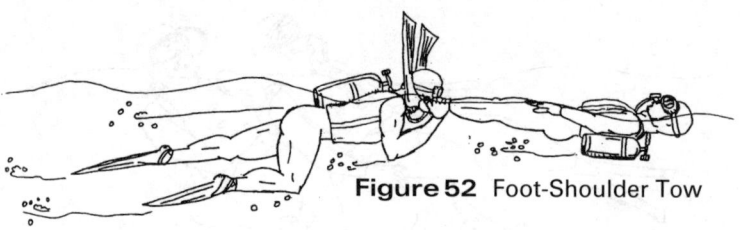

Figure 52 Foot-Shoulder Tow

Rescue Breathing

Delivering rescue breaths to a victim in water can be done in a variety of ways, but effective chest compressions are not feasible while trying to tow a diver. The rescuer should therefore not waste time trying to establish if there is a pulse. The rescuer should be aware of the likelihood of the victim vomiting after aspiration. Using an instrument (pocket mask or snorkel) to perform rescue breathing may help protect the rescuer from the victim's body fluids. The rescuer can be behind the victim's back or at their side depending on the type of rescue breathing being delivered. More than one rescuer improves the delivery of rescue breathing while generating a more rapid tow. Full CPR can be administered once the victim is out of the water. Removing the victim's weights will allow for better buoyancy and less drag during the tow. One may consider removing the victim's air tank from their BCD harness to further improve buoyancy and diminish drag while towing. Removing the rescuer's weights will allow for better buoyancy and allow the rescuer to deliver breaths to the victim with greater ease. The rescuer may keep their tank and BCD or hand it off to a fellow rescuer to allow for less cumbersome equipment during delivery of rescue breathing to the victim.

Rescue breathing is begun by making sure the vest is nearfully inflated for maximum buoyancy. The vest must be checked to be sure that the diver has no restriction to expansion of their chest. If the vest has a poor fit that compresses the chest it can be unsnapped or loosened. In rough weather the vest may be loosened, but unsnapping the vest could increase the risk of the victim falling out, especially when a small individual is wearing a large-fitting vest. The victim's weights are dropped and the rescuer removes the victim's mask and regulator. The rescuer may elect to keep his or her own mask on, especially in rough weather.

Mouth-to-mouth rescue breathing can be done effectively only from beside the victim. The rescuer delivering breaths from beside the victim during a tow should place his or her arm closest to the victim's feet under the victim's axilla (underarm) and around behind the victim's head (Do-Si-Do position) (See Figure 53 for In-water mouth to mouth rescue breathing). The hair or hood is grasped to tilt the victim's head back. While pinching the nose with the other hand, the rescuer delivers breaths every five seconds. The rescuer must attempt to maintain an active tow during the delivery of rescue breathing to get the victim to shore or the boat as expeditiously as possible.

Performing rescue breathing with a pocket mask can be done in a similar fashion as when delivering mouth-to-mouth or may be done with the rescuer behind the victims' head (See Figure 54 for Mouth-to-mask rescue breathing). In this manner the rescuer holds the victim's head and jaw with both hands. The head is tilted back toward the rescuer. The pocket mask is held firmly covering the victim's nose and mouth with the thumbs and index fingers, and breaths are delivered while the rescuer continually swims backward toward shore or the vessel. This method of delivering breaths allows for a more efficient and quicker tow than mouth-to-mouth or mouth-to-mask from the victim's side.

Rescue breathing with a snorkel is performed with the rescuer behind the victim's head (See Figure 55 for Mouth-to-Snorkel Rescue Breaths). The snorkel mouthpiece is held firmly in the victim's mouth with the rescuer's hand. The ring finger is used to hold the victim's jaw. The middle finger is used to help the victim's upper lip form a

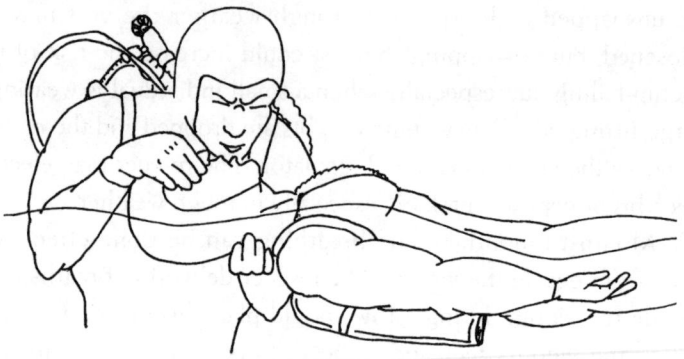

Figure 53 In-water Mouth-to-Mouth Rescue Breathing.

Figure 54 In-Water Mouth-to-Mask Rescue Breathing.

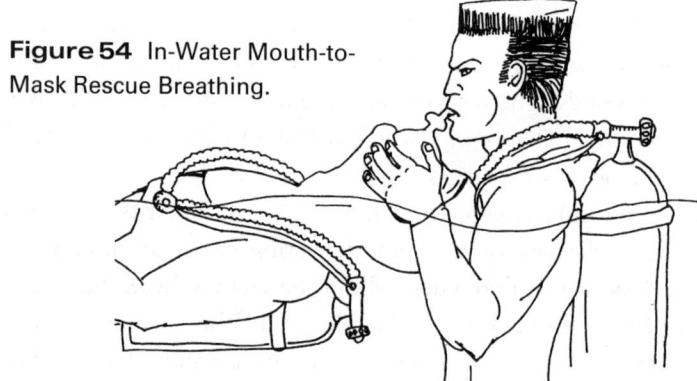

seal on the snorkel, and the index finger and thumb are used to pinch the nostrils closed. The head is held tilted back and the rescuer delivers ventilation by blowing into the end of the snorkel from behind the victim while towing them. The advantage of this method of rescue breathing is that the rescuer does not have to elevate himself or herself out of the water as far to deliver the breaths and is therefore less fatigued and will allow for a faster tow. The disadvantage is that the length of the snorkel adds to the dead space of the victim's respiratory system. This is a minor disadvantage. The newer snorkels with purge or flood valves will not allow for this type of rescue breathing.

Exit with a Victim

After the victim has been towed to shore, the rescuer may find it much easier and lighter to remove the victim's gear and their own gear in order to exit with the victim. A conscious victim should assist in their exit by walking if possible. An unconscious victim must be lifted out of the water or carried out of the water.

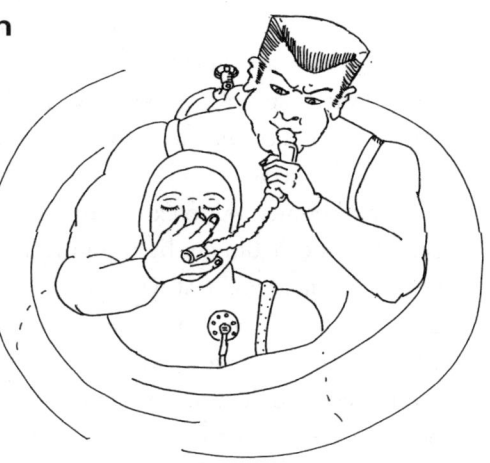

Figure 55 In-Water Mouth-to-Snorkel Rescue Breathing.

The more numerous the rescuers, the less dangerous and difficult the exit becomes. Recruiting others along shore to help is a significant benefit to getting a victim out safely. Two people can usually handle a victim by supporting them with the victim's arms around the rescuer's shoulders (See Figure 56 for Rescuer Exit with Victim).

Along shore, the methods of exit for a lone rescuer and their victim depend on the water movements, the bottom composition and topography, the abilities of the rescuer, and the size of the victim. A strong rescuer and a light victim may allow for carrying the victim out in their arms, the Cradle or Arm carry (See Figure 58 for Cradle carry exit with victim). The Fireman's carry is where the victim is swung across the rescuer's shoulders (See Figure 57 for Fireman carry exit with victim), and the Saddleback carry is where the victim is stretched across the rescuer's back (See Figure 60 for Saddleback carry exit with victim). Both of these carrying styles require a relatively strong rescuer and a manageably proportioned victim. The smaller rescuer with a large victim may use the Packstrap carry as the preferred method where the victim is draped over the rescuer's back and their arms are pulled over the rescuer's shoulders (See Figure 59 for Packstrap carry exit with victim). In shallow water, the packstrap carry is the easiest way to carry a victim toward shore unless CPR is being performed.

Another method to exit with a larger victim than one can carry is to drag the victim out by the arms (Hand-Pull exit) (See Figure 61 below for Hand-Pull exit with victim). A small rescuer can usually carry out a large victim if the rescuer carries them on their back while exiting on hands and knees. In heavy surge and large waves, the rescuer should exit on hands and knees as soon as the water becomes shallow enough to do so. Using the surge and wave to make progress is only frustrated by the back-wash one experiences as the waves wash back out. Avoidance of coral, rocks, or other obstacles is important in strong surge or large waves.

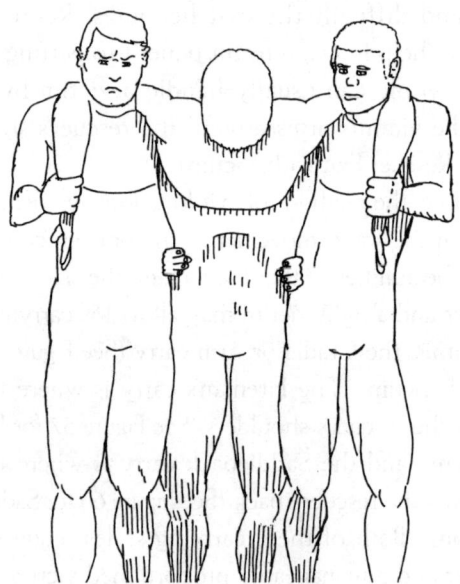

Figure 56 Two-Rescuer Exit

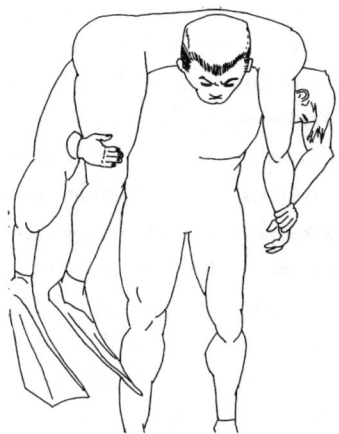

Figure 57 Fireman Carry

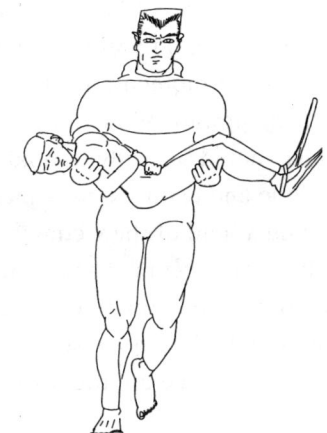

Figure 58 Cradle or Arm Carry

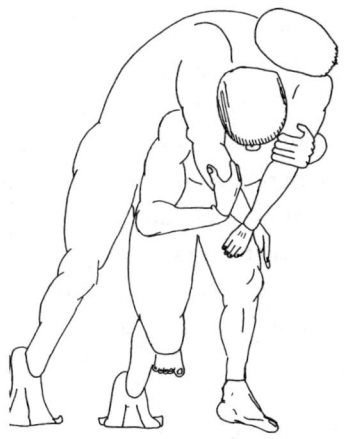

Figure 59 Packstrap Carry

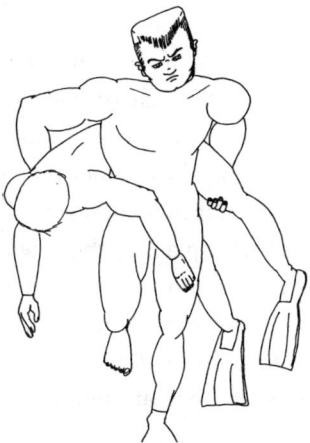

Figure 60 Saddleback Carry

Exiting onto a boat is done with all hands on deck assisting. The crew should grasp the hands of the victim and haul the victim up. By momentarily letting the victim sink slightly before heaving upward allows for a more effective lift. The rescuer in the water should be ready to hold the victim should they fall back in. If alone and exiting onto a pier, the rescuer is to exit while maintaining a hold of the victim (See Figures 62-65 for exit onto pier with victim). The victim's hands can be placed on the pier (or platform of a boat) while the rescuer puts their hand on top of the victim's hands while lifting himself or herself onto the pier (or boat swim platform). Once up, the rescuer can hold the hands of the victim and pull them up to lay them on the pier. A small rescuer and a large victim may require the rescuer to push the victim underwater momentarily to get some momentum to be able to lift the victim out onto the pier or swim platform.

A rescuer raising a victim onto a tall pier or dock will require assistance from someone on the dock. A line can be wrapped around the chest of the victim to raise them (See Figure 66 below for lifting victim with rope). The rope is wrapped around the victim's chest under the armpits and raised quickly to prevent the victim from slipping out. If the victim's arms can be secured by placing them within their belt, trunks, or expose suit zipper it may help keep their arms from extending upward, preventing the diver from slipping out of the rope that is wrapped around their chest.

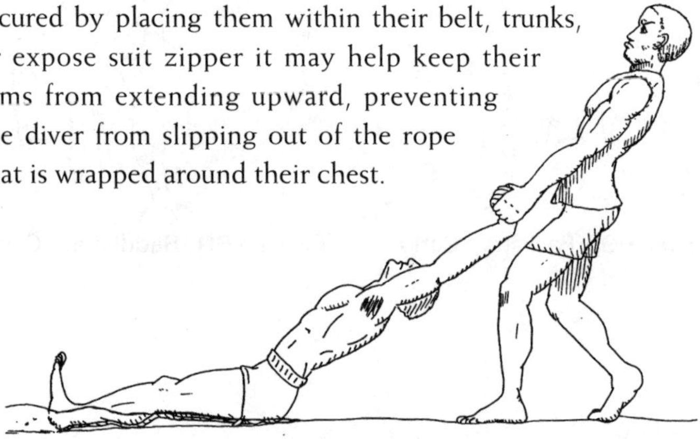

Figure 61 Hand-Pull Exit

SURFACE EMERGENCIES

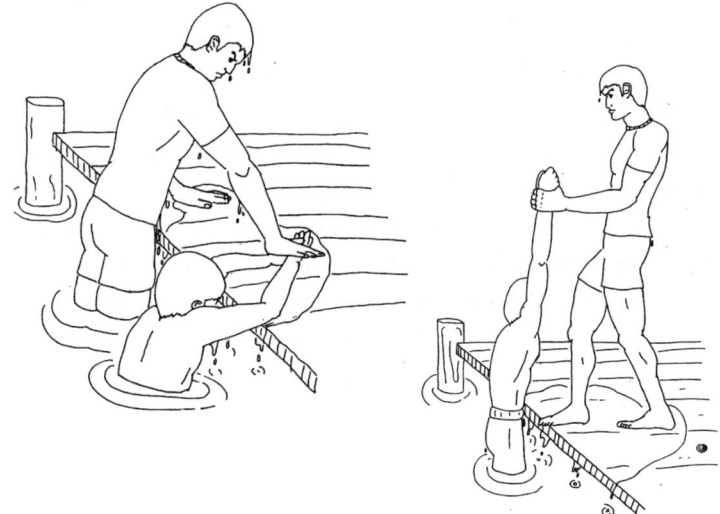

Figure 62 Rescuer lifts himself out with hand on victim's hand.

Figure 63 Lift victim up by the arms.

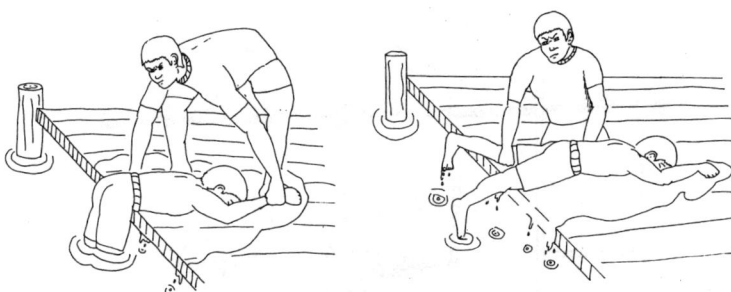

Figure 64 Lay victim on pier with hips flexed over edge of pier.

Figure 65 Pull victim's legs onto pier.

A ladder at the edge of a pier may be useful for a large rescuer to carry a light victim up (See Figure 67 for exit by ladder with victim). This can be done by placing the victim's legs straddled over one of the rescuer's thigh, and the victim's arms around the neck and over the shoulders of the rescuer. The rescuer needs to keep the knee of the leg supporting the victim somewhat bent during the entire climb. The rescuer must assess the strength and integrity of the ladder to be sure it will support the combined weight of the victim and rescuer as they climb to the pier. Once near the top, the rescuer can lay the victim on their back on the pier when the victim's buttocks are able to clear the floor of the pier.

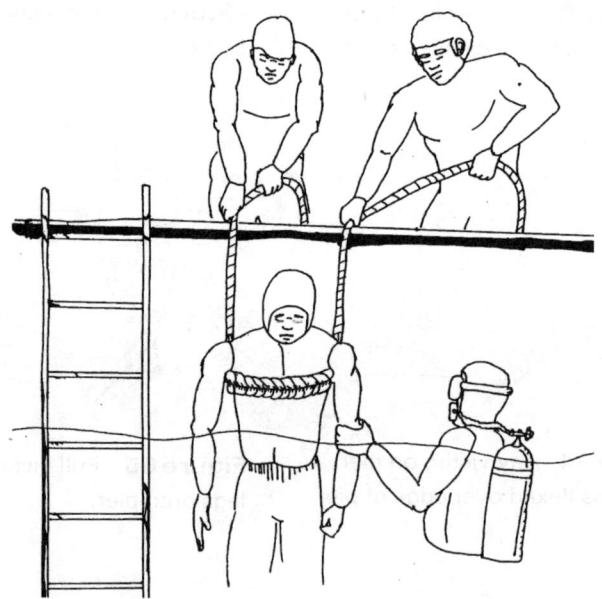

Figure 66 Lifting a victim onto a pier with a rope wrapped around the chest.

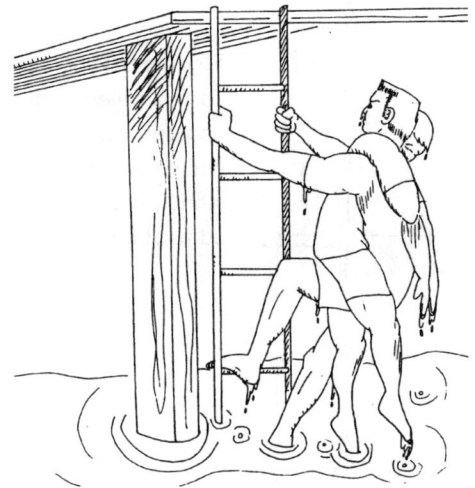

Figure 67 Exiting with a victim straddled over the rescuers thigh.

A blanket or tarp can be lowered from a pier in order to perform a roll-up technique in order to raise a victim from the water to the pier (See Figures 68-69 for Lifting victim with tarp). Ropes are tied to the two ends of the blanket that are lowered to the water level. The two ends that remain on the pier are stepped on by the rescuers on the pier to prevent them from slipping off the pier. The victim is placed lengthwise along the edge of the blanket that is in the water and the blanket is pulled under and around them. Pulling up on the ropes will roll the victim up to the pier.

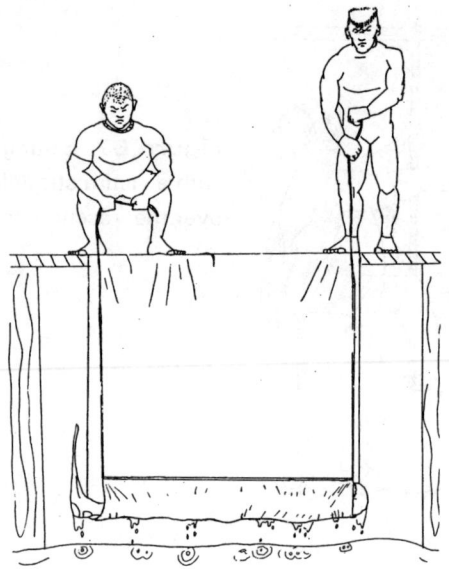

Figure 68
Tarp is rolled under and around victim while rescuers stand on upper edge of tarp.

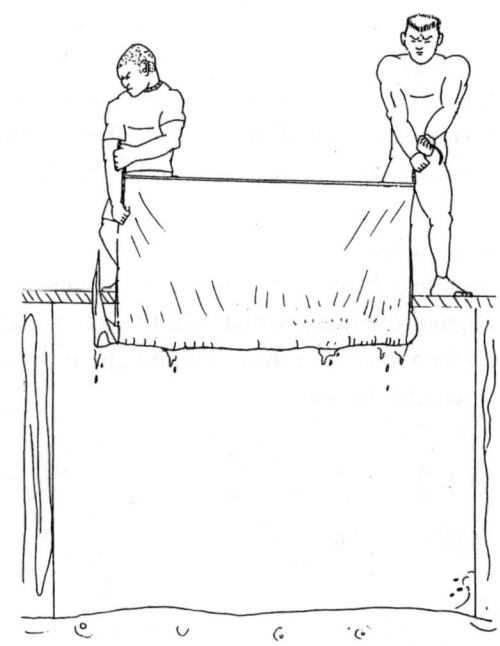

Figure 69
Tarp is pulled up with the ropes and the victim is rolled up to the pier.

CHAPTER SIX

Boating Emergencies

Management of any emergency on a vessel needs coordinated action of all passengers and crew onboard. The captain is to be in charge of emergencies and coordinating activities on the vessel. He or she may designate duties as required or depending on the experience or expertise of the crew or passengers. The captain's familiarity with the vessel, its equipment, and its capabilities makes him or her the optimal individual to be in charge of emergency management decisions. The boat captain should remain onboard the vessel at all times unless extraneous circumstances dictate otherwise. It is not a rare occurrence for an anchor to drag or the mooring line to fail, causing the vessel to drift. Depending on the current and/or the wind, the drift of the vessel may be faster than individuals in the water can swim. If the captain is not onboard a major problem may develop.

Lightning

Lightning strikes to a vessel may cause vessel damage and personal injury or death. The electrical current from a bolt of lightning may exceed 100 million volts of electrical power and exceed 50,000 degrees Fahrenheit (28,000 degrees C). About 50% of lightning-related injuries involve recreational activities and water-related strikes may approach 40% in certain geographical areas. A vessel is at particular risk in open water because of the lack of other tall structures that would compete with the vessel to attract the lightning bolt.

The best protection to a vessel and its passengers is to avoid boating during weather that is conducive to the risk of lightning. The second best protection is to have a lightning protection system onboard. A lightning protection system neither decreases nor increases the likelihood of a lightning strike. These systems are merely designed to attract the lightning bolt to the air terminal (vertical conductor) and direct the current through a copper wire to a hull plate where the current is then dissipated into the body of water. Having a lightning protection system may avoid or at least decrease the likelihood of damage. The copper wire that conducts the current from a lightning strike may vaporize from overheating. For this reason, the heavier the size of the wire the better. It is recommended that vessels have #4 copper wire or heavier. The recommended size for the grounding plate is at least one inch (2.54 cm) wide and twelve feet (3.7 meters) long.

When the conditions are favorable to the likelihood of a lightning strike, the crew and passengers may elect to place their life vests on. In order to avoid becoming the object directly struck by the bolt of lightning, everyone may enter the cabin and stay off deck. Staying away from metal railings and electrical equipment that is wired to the main circuits of the vessel may protect against electrocution if a lightning bolt strikes the vessel. Prevent contact with faucets and metal fittings, which may include the wheel if made of metal.

If a bolt of lightning has struck one's vessel, personnel must survey the vessel and check all passengers for the proper head count and any injuries. Damage to the vessel may include complete meltdown of the vessel's electronics, explosion of the fuel, a vaporized vessel antennae, blowout of the through-hull fittings, and large holes blown through the hull. Fire, loss of electrical and engine power, and taking on water are likely results of the above. Injuries may include burns, seizures, cardiac and pulmonary arrest, and death. The treatment is directed at the specific injuries sustained and repairs are prioritized by the risk of losing ship or passengers. Teams should be simultaneously assigned to rescue, treat, and repair the highest priority passenger threats, injuries, and vessel breakdowns. The crew may need to be assigned tasks for checking the integrity of the hull, electrical systems, and engines. Specific injuries and damage to the vessel are managed as required by the circumstances. A man overboard situation is simultaneously attended to. Calling for help sooner rather than later is wiser. A hand-held radio or phone may be indispensable if there is complete power failure of the vessel's electronics.

Lost at Sea

The best defense against being lost at sea is attentiveness to one's coarse, speed, and time as well as a thorough knowledge of the local waterways and a full set of charts for the region. The best plan to deal with being lost at sea is having had a set departure and return time, a set destination, and a responsible individual who is not onboard who will initiate a search if the vessel has not returned within a reasonable period of time. If cruising out of visibility of land, the operator or captain should plot his or her course and calculate their position using proper plotting techniques.

A captain with the proper vessel electronics would have a GPS (global positioning system) or Loran system aboard and should never need to worry about being lost. Having a hand-held or battery-powered system would prevent being lost in case of a power failure. Every vessel needs a compass and ship to shore radio for this eventuality. An EPIRB (Emergency Position Indicating Radio Beacon) can transmit a signal that can be detected up to 300 miles (480 Km) away. These units can be activated manually or automatically if submerged. Once activated, these units should remain on until the battery is totally discharged.

The first measure to take should be attempting contact with another vessel or local authorities. A ship to shore radio has only a limited distance of transmission but bypassing vessels may be able to pickup the signal and offer assistance and coordinates within a fifteen mile radius. Radio transmissions for help are to be sent on the hour and every half-hour to conserve the battery. If contact is made information is given pertaining to the name, size, and color of the vessel, the number of passengers, the nature of your distress, assistance required, the last known location, and the time since being at the last known location.

If lost and another vessel is seen at a distance, contact may be attempted with any of a large variety of devices. Flares, lights, mirrors, fire (smoke), dye, horn sounding, radio, bell ringing, flags, and waving of the arms are the most frequent methods of signaling to another vessel that there is trouble aboard. Use signaling devices carefully and in the most productive manner. Try to use the reusable signaling devices first (mirror, lights, radio, horn, etc.) and save the others (i.e., flares) for when they may be best visualized. An airplane will be able to sight a signal two to three times further (thirty to forty miles or fifty to sixty-five Km) than a vessel (twelve to fifteen miles or nineteen to twenty-four Km) due to the curvature of the Earth. Use reusable signaling devices as soon as another vessel is sighted or a plane is heard (even if it is not seen). Save the flares or smoke signals for when the plane or vessel is at its closest position in their path.

If you are truly lost at sea and have no instrumentation (GPS or Loran) to find your position you can determine latitude and longitude using the sun and your watch. One must be within 60 degrees north and 60 degrees south of the equator. Exceptions are dates between March 11 through 13, and September 13 through October 2. The concept behind the calculation of latitude is that depending on the latitude, the sun will take a known specific amount of time to cross the sky on a specific date. The concept behind calculating longitude is that the Earth's spin on its axis is at a constant velocity. We know that the Earth spins one degree longitude every four minutes. Since zero longitude is in Greenwich, England, one can determine the number of degrees of longitude away from Greenwich by how many hours and minutes it takes the sun to get from directly over Greenwich to directly over your position.

In order to find your latitude use the following steps:

1. Use your timepiece to time the exact length of day from the instant the sun is visible on the eastern horizon to the instant it disappears on the western horizon.

2. Using the Nomogram in Figure 70, draw a straight line from the length of the day at the bottom to the date at the top of the Nomogram.

3. The latitude is where the line intersects the vertical center latitude line.

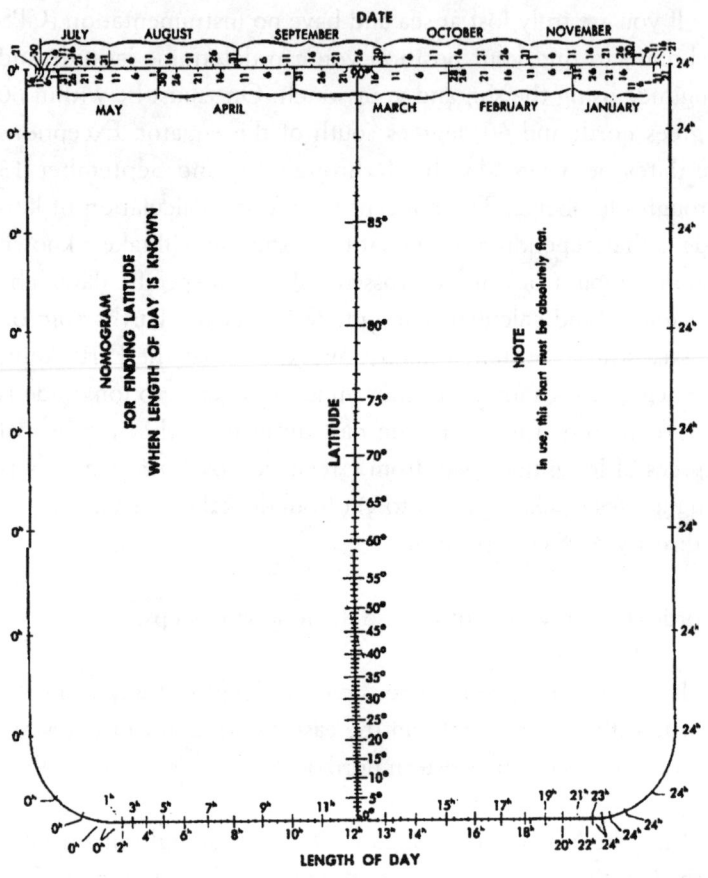

Figure 70 Latitude Nomogram

In order to find longitude use the following steps:
1. Convert Daylight Savings time (if being used) to Standard time.
2. Convert time to military time.
3. Establish local noontime. Noon is exactly halfway between sunrise and sunset. Divide total hours and minutes of daylight by two.
4. Convert local noontime to Greenwich time. Use World Time Zone Chart in Table 10 on page 175 to find the number of hours to add or subtract for conversion.

TABLE 10
WORLD TIME ZONE CHART

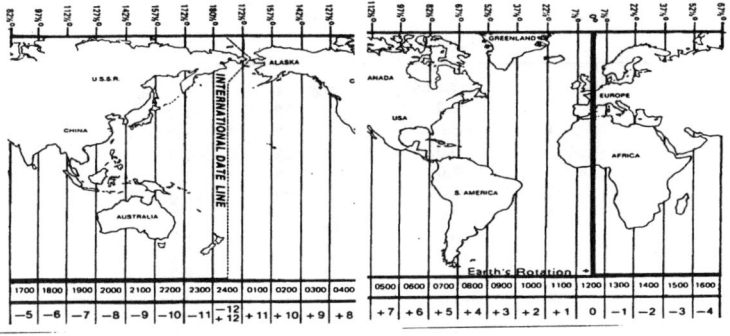

5. Adjust time of "apparent" noon. Use Date/Time Equation Chart in Table 11 on page 176 to find the number of minutes to add or subtract for adjustment.
6. Calculate the difference between Greenwich noon and the Greenwich time of local apparent noon. The difference in time will determine the number of hours and minutes.
7. Calculate the number of degrees longitude you are away from Greenwich, England using the following formula:
   a. Every hour equals 15 degrees.
   b. Every four minutes equals 1 degree.
   c. Every minute of time equals 15 navigational minutes of longitude.
   d. Use fractions of a degree within your calculation and convert to navigational minutes. There are 60 minutes per degree (do not confuse navigational minutes with minutes of time).

TABLE 11
APPARENT TIME CONVERSION CHART

Date	Eq. of Time*	Date	Eq. of Time*
Jan. 1	−3.5 min.	Aug. 4	−6.0 min.
2	−4.0	12	−5.0
4	−5.0	17	−4.0
7	−6.0	22	−3.0
9	−7.0	26	−2.0
12	−8.0	29	−1.0
14	−9.0	Sept. 1	0.0
17	−10.0	5	+1.0
20	−11.0	8	+2.0
24	−12.0	10	+3.0
28	−13.0	13	+4.0
Feb. 4	−14.0	16	+5.0
13	−14.3	19	+6.0
19	−14.0	22	+7.0
28	−13.0	25	+8.0
Mar. 4	−12.0	28	+9.0
8	−11.0	Oct. 1	+10.0
12	−10.0	4	+11.0
16	−9.0	7	+12.0
19	−8.0	11	+13.0
22	−7.0	15	+14.0
26	−6.0	20	+15.0
29	−5.0	27	+16.0
Apr. 1	−4.0	Nov. 4	+16.4
5	−3.0	11	+16.0
8	−2.0	17	+15.0
12	−1.0	22	+14.0
16	0.0	25	+13.0
20	+1.0	28	+12.0
25	+2.0	Dec. 1	+11.0
May 2	+3.0	4	+10.0
14	+3.8	6	+9.0
28	+3.0	9	+8.0
June 4	+2.0	11	+7.0
9	+1.0	13	+6.0
14	0.0	15	+5.0
19	−1.0	17	+4.0
23	−2.0	19	+3.0
28	−3.0	21	+2.0
July 3	−4.0	23	+1.0
9	−5.0	25	0.0
18	−6.0	27	−1.0
27	−6.6	29	−2.0
		31	−3.0

*Add plus to time and subtract from time to get apparent time.

Taking on Water

A variety of circumstances may lead to taking on water. A disconnection or leak in a hose, an open valve, high waves, open hatches, a defective stuffing box, collision, and a multitude of other problems can cause a vessel to take on water that may overcome the bilge capacity. Every vessel should be equipped with an emergency leak repair kit. This kit should have as a minimum a variety of sizes of wooden corks, a tube of underwater putty, rags, and duct tape.

When taking on water, the first responsibility is to the passengers and crew. Life jackets should be donned immediately and all personnel are asked to go to the upper deck. Life rafts should be deployed and ready to be boarded if abandoning ship is necessary. If divers are on board they may consider donning their wet suits to add buoyancy and insulation if prolonged exposure may occur. The captain or vessel operator should assess the need to immediately contact the Coast Guard or nearby vessels.

Investigation of all hoses, valves, and stuffing boxes should be done in an expeditious manner if possible. If the bilge is completely flooded, this may be impossible and abandoning ship may be the only option left. If, however, inspection can be done of the bilge and the source of the leak is identified, there may be a chance to repair or slow down the leak. The bilge pump should be activated if not already in use. All valves responsible for any leakage should be closed. Locating the source of the leak may be difficult. Visually inspecting the hull may prove fruitless, but feeling for the leak with one's hand or foot may identify the inward flow of water. This can also be done behind obstructions that cannot be visualized.

When working in the bilge the engines should be shut down. However, if the leak can be slowed and the vessel is still taking on water that may be above the capacity of the bilge pump, the engines may be converted into a bilge pump. The valve for the water intake for the engine cooling system is to be shut off. The water intake hose for the engine is disconnected from the hull and placed into the water in the deepest possible aspect of the bilge. When the engines are restarted the engine cooling system will suck the water from the bilge and blow it out as the vessel heads for harbor.

Leaks from hoses may be handled in a few ways. Hoses with a small or large hole may be temporarily repaired by tightly wrapping them with a generous amount of duct tape. Wooded corks can also be used to cork a small leak in hoses and secured with the duct tape. This may not stop the leak completely but may reduce the leak to within the capacity of the bilge pump. Closing the valve of the hose may solve the leak problem. If, however, the hose is part of the engine cooling system, duct tape or a cork will still allow water to flow to the engine (although reduced if a cork is used) in order to reach the shore or harbor.

A small hole in the hull may similarly be plugged with a wooded cork (preferably from the outside). Application of underwater putty around the cork will help seal the opening. Leaking cracks may be temporarily sealed with application of underwater putty, preferably from the outside. Larger holes in the hull have little chance of remedy due to the limited resources and time that the crew may have at hand. The crew may attempt to take cloth wrapped in plastic and stuff it into a larger hole covered with duct tape from the outside in an attempt to decrease the water flow. This may buy time to allow the Coast Guard to arrive and rescue the crew and passengers, but this will usually not be strong enough to withstand the forces during cruising back to shore. Wrapping a strong, water-resistant tarp on the outside of the hull and using ropes tied to the corners of the tarp to stretch it over the hull may help seal the leak (See Figure 71 for Covering Hull with Tarp). Make a knot at each corner of the tarp to prevent the rope from slipping off the tarp. Pull the ropes tight and secure them to the cleats on

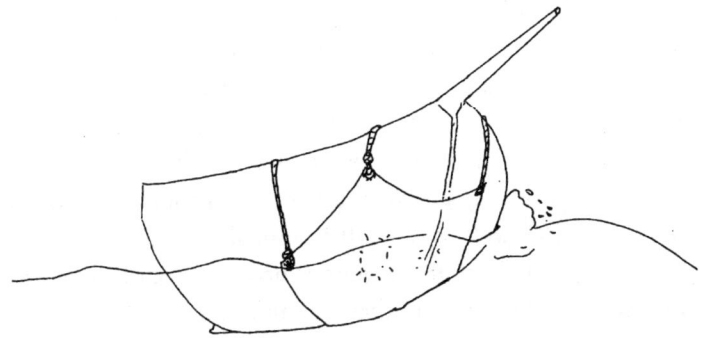

Figure 71 Tying a waterproof tarp around hull keeping leading edge above the water line to seal a large hole.

the side of the vessel to hold the tarp snug on the hull. The water pressure will help hold the tarp in place even while cruising if the leak is near the bow. If cruising with the tarp on the bow is attempted, be sure the leading edge of the tarp is above the waterline to prevent the water from getting under the tarp and pulling it off the hull. This will not be effective while cruising if the leak is at the center or stern of the hull but may slow the leak while the vessel is stationary.

Leakage from the stuffing box that seals the propeller shaft as it exits the bilge can be corrected with the proper wrench. On many vessels the stuffing box tightens in opposite directions on the starboard and port engines. Tightening the stuffing box may require an intense force and will require the repair person to climb into the bilge. The engines and all electrical circuits should be shut off to avoid injury to personnel during the repair.

If foul weather and high waves are the cause of taking on water, the vessel operator may consider changing the vessel's angle of approach to the waves. Shutting all hatches and windows may help the bilge from flooding. Adjusting the vessel's speed may prevent taking on waves over the transom or submarining of the bow as the vessel comes over a large wave. Foul weather may continue to worsen and the water line may continue to rise from progressive flooding, causing a cycle of worsening circumstances. Radio contacts with the Coast Guard for assistance, sooner rather than later, is the wisest course of action if taking on water during a storm or angry seas. Electric and manual bilge pumps are to be used as well as any other modality that will assist in eliminating water. Care to prevent a man overboard situation is of utmost importance within these circumstances.

Collision

The captain of any vessel involved in a collision is always the individual ultimately responsible for the collision. When two vessels collide, the operators or captains of both vessels are considered at fault. Following proper procedures as described in the unified rules of the road for vessel operations will lessen the likelihood of collision. Observance of good seamanship, proper vessel communication, and timely action by the vessel operators will usually ensure safe boating.

Whenever two or more vessels are in proximity a risk of collision exists. The unified rules suggest that a vessel operator take action in ample time and with due regard to good seamanship. Any alteration of course and/or speed should be large enough to be obvious to the other vessels (i.e., avoiding a succession of small changes in course and/or speed). Check and recheck the effectiveness of one's actions and the other vessel's actions until the other vessels are clear. One may need to slow or stop one's vessel, or even reverse the engines. Sound the proper signals of intention when in sight of another vessel and follow the prescribed rules for meeting, crossing, and overtaking another vessel.

There is a hierarchy designated for determining the "privileged" vessel. This hierarchy specifies who has the right of way.

The vessel most privileged is always the vessel being overtaken. All other vessels must stay clear of any vessel they are overtaking. The vessel being overtaken has the responsibility of maintaining its speed and course in order to allow the other vessel to predictably anticipate its movements. Vessels not under command (vessels having difficulty with power or steering) are next in order. Vessels restricted in maneuverability (vessels restricted due to water depth or bridge height, for example) are next in order of privilege. Vessels engaged in fishing are the next in the pecking order. Sailing vessels are the next privileged vessels followed by power-driven vessels (sailboats that are under power are considered power-driven vessels and must give way to other sailboats). Seaplanes are the least privileged and must keep clear of all other vessels.

The most common causes of vessel collision are inattention or carelessness, improper lookout, obstructed view, speeding, navigational error, and violation of navigation rules. Alcohol use is a major contributor to many of the above collision factors. Most collisions occur around midday on weekends.

When a collision occurs, a rapid assessment of the situation must be made. Several factors must be immediately investigated, including the risk of further damage or taking on water, spillage of flammable liquids, fire, injuries, and accounting of all passengers and crew. All personnel should be required to don life jackets. Life rafts should be deployed and if necessary personnel asked to abandon ship. All injuries are to be attended to and anyone who has fallen overboard is to immediately be rescued. Emergency personnel are to be contacted immediately (Coast Guard and EMS).

Abandoning Ship

Abandoning ship is a last resort to a maritime emergency. Many vessels can withstand substantial damage and not sink.

Even if a vessel takes on a large quantity of water, many vessels are made to float at the surface and not sink to the bottom. But passengers should not wait until the very end to deploy the raft and have provisions ready to abandon ship.

Immediately after a significant problem has been encountered that can lead to a need to abandon ship, all passengers and crew need to don life jackets. The crew or designated passengers should then be assigned and simultaneously directed to send an SOS, assess injuries, and assess vessel damage. Next, the crew and designated passengers are assigned to begin to treat injuries, attempt to repair the vessel if possible, and to deploy the raft if appropriate. Deploying the raft is done sooner rather than later in case there is a problem with the automatic deployment and manual deployment is needed, which can take much longer.

Launching the life raft on the leeward side of the damaged vessel has several advantages. The main vessel will protect the raft from the wind while repair of the vessel may be attempted or passengers are boarding. Provisions placed in the raft may be more protected from the wind and waves. When the main vessel sinks, the life raft will not get blown into the sinking vessel, avoiding damage to the raft or getting it entangled with the sinking vessel. Floating objects from the sinking vessel that may be usable may be easier to salvage. Before launching the raft, be sure that the line is secured to both the raft and the vessel. Tie the line so that it can be lengthened without having to untie it.

Boarding the life raft may be done from the vessel or the water while trying to keep as much water out of the raft as possible. The first individual on the raft should be a strong crew member to assist and coordinate the other individuals boarding the raft. The second person on the raft should be stationed at the painter armed with a knife and ready to cut the line securing the raft to the sinking vessel. The last person to board the raft should be responsible for passing the provisions that have not already been loaded onto the raft. After the last individual has boarded, the raft's line is let out as much as possible but not cut. The vessel may not sink and it may be more visible to a search crew than a small raft. Letting out as much line as possible will dampen the tugging on the raft from the effect of the waves on the vessel. Should the vessel actually sink, cut the line immediately as one feels the pull on the raft.

If there is more than one raft, they need to be tied together at a safe distance apart depending on the weather and water conditions. Tying them together from the start may be one's only opportunity to keep the rafts in proximity of each other. Dividing the rations equally between rafts is the wisest plan, placing half of each provision in each raft. If, for instance, all the drinking water is placed in one raft and the rafts separate or that one raft capsizes, the individuals in the other raft or the whole group will be out of provisions.

Provisions need to be loaded onto the raft in order of their importance to survival. It is important to remember that passengers are the priority, not provisions. Overloading a raft can jeopardize the whole group. Provisions need to be rationed. Most healthy individuals should be able to tolerate no food and very little water if any for the first day.

Provisions needed on a raft are the raft repair kit, sea anchors (two or three), knife, bailing container, lights, flares, mirror, GPS, and radio. These items are the most important for raft maintenance, positioning, and communication attempts. Water, non-perishable food, sunscreen, first aid kit, and needed medication are also high on the priority list. These are basic essentials for survival. A multitude of other less important items may be salvaged from the sinking vessel (including wet suits) that may make a stay on a raft more comfortable and survivable.

Man Overboard

When a passenger or crew member falls off a vessel and into the water unintentionally it is considered a "man overboard" condition. Boarding and disembarkment at a slip or dock is a particularly vulnerable time when this can occur, especially with passengers who are not familiar or accustomed to boating. Many boats have railings that need to be climbed over to step onto the boat or dock. Boats have a natural tendency to sway and move towards and away from the dock. A passenger should first step onto the deck of the boat outside the railing, then step over the railing with the other leg to prevent them from being pulled away from the dock with one leg caught over a railing should the boat move away from the dock. To disembark, the passenger is to first step over the railing with both feet, then step across to the dock for the same reason.

Falling into the water while the vessel is tied to the dock can be quite hazardous because of the risk of injury due to striking the boat, the dock, or both on the way down. The risk of a crush injury is quite high if the boat swings toward the dock while the passenger is falling or hanging between the boat and the dock. The risk of a man overboard is even higher when there are transfers of passengers from one vessel onto another vessel while in open water. In this case there are two swaying or rocking platforms that must be taken into consideration. The difficulty in this maneuver is made much more hazardous in rough waters.

Rough water with high waves and inexperience increases the risks of a man overboard while cruising. Passengers need to be instructed on how to move about a boat and where and how to hold on while walking from the stern to the bow and vice versa. Attentiveness to one's passengers is of utmost importance, especially in rough water. The use of life jackets by passengers may be seriously considered, especially for young, elderly, and inexperienced boaters.

A man overboard at the bow while underway can be much more hazardous than from the stern or the sides of the boat because of the potential for a propeller injury. Head, spine, and other potentially life-threatening injuries can occur from striking the swim platform or lower decks while falling. The victim may lose consciousness from a variety of causes, including the possibility that losing consciousness may be the reason they fell in to begin with. It is therefore necessary to think ahead when attempting a rescue of a man overboard. As soon as a man overboard situation has been identified, one or more individuals should immediately begin preparing to enter the water by donning exposure suits and life vests to execute a rescue.

A passenger who is witnessed falling off allows the captain to know immediately and the benefit of knowing exactly where the victim is located. This also affords the rescuers the benefit of identifying potential associated injuries due to the specifics of the fall. If the victim is on the surface and conscious a life ring can be thrown to them immediately. If the victim is not seen, a marker buoy should be thrown in immediately to mark the site of the victim's last whereabouts. If the victim is not seen to surface, an immediate underwater search is conducted with all qualified divers working in buddy teams.

If the victim was not witnessed falling overboard, the vessel must be turned around and a search is to be initiated. An estimate of the elapsed time from the last sighting of the missing passenger from other passengers and the vessel's speed can determine the distance within which the victim may be found. Wave height, current, tide, and wind will be factors that may influence the scope of the search area. Calling for emergency personnel should be done immediately.

The course the vessel takes during a search is usually along the same course that was already traveled. The water usually maintains a trail of the vessel's course due to the wake, and bubbles within the water from the propellers makes backtracking fairly straightforward. Even if there is a current, the trail will be carried by the current. The scope of the search should include the area between the vessel's trail carried by the current and the exact navigational coarse taken. Extreme care must be taken not to run over an unconscious victim at or just under the surface. All available personnel are to act as lookouts with all available binoculars. The lookouts are to be positioned at the bow to search ahead and the stern to look behind, as well as the port (left), and starboard (right) of the vessel. The higher the vantage point of the lookouts the better their view, especially in high waves. Polarized sunglasses may help reduce glare and improve visualization at and just below the surface of the water.

The use of life jackets with lights by passengers at night makes a man overboard scenario significantly less bleak. Without the benefit of a light, it would be quite unlikely to find an unconscious victim at or just below the surface in the dark. Recruiting professional help as quickly as possible may increase the chances of a successful search and recovery after dark. The use of a bright spotlight on the front of the vessel and powerful flashlights by all the lookouts may increase the possibility of spotting the victim.

Once the victim is spotted, at least one lookout should try and maintain constant visual contact with them. This can be difficult in high waves. When approaching a victim the vessel should be in complete control. Approaching the victim should be done at slow speed and on the windward side (side from where wind is coming from) to keep the vessel from drifting away from the victim. The vessel should be pulled up alongside the victim. Once near the victim, the vessel should be stopped dead and the gears placed in neutral. Rough waters and high waves increase the risk of further injury to the victim and the rescuers in the water from being struck by the hull of the boat. In this circumstance, the vessel may approach the victim from the leeward side (side that the wind is blowing toward) to prevent the vessel from being blown over the victim and striking them with the hull.

A conscious victim should have a life ring with an attached buoyant line heaved slightly past them and slightly to the windward side, not at them. An unconscious victim should have a rescuer enter the water wearing a life jacket and in possession of a life ring with a line whose end is secured by the boat crew to pull them in with. The rescuer can then swim to the victim and they can both be pulled to the boat by the line. Once alongside the vessel, a second line can be lowered and wrapped around the victim's chest, under the arms, in order to hoist them onto the vessel (See Figure 66 on page 166 for lifting victim with rope).

Once onboard, the victim is to be assessed for injuries, hypothermia, and aspiration. The appropriate treatment including CPR must be initiated at once and continued until trained medical personnel arrive.

Fire

A fire onboard a vessel is a true emergency and involves a threat to both the vessel and passengers. It must be extinguished immediately and all measures must be taken to prepare for a potential abandonment of the ship. The risk to the vessel is not only from flame but also from the potential for explosion. The risks to passengers and crew are not only from flame and explosion, but also from the dangers of smoke inhalation. All passengers are to be moved to the safest area of the vessel (usually on deck) and life vests need to be donned at once. Deployment of rafts must be considered, as the circumstances require. Calling for help and mobilizing the EMS also needs to be considered depending on the circumstances, before power is lost or the vessel sinks.

A fire requires four essential ingredients: fuel, heat, oxygen, and a chain reaction. Eliminate any of these elements and a fire will die out. There are four basic fire classifications. They are classified by the burning fuel. Wood, cloth, and other things that produce A̲sh cause type A̲ fires. B̲ottled fuels such as gasoline, alcohol, butane, and others cause type B̲ fires. Electrical C̲urrent causes type C̲ fires. Flammable metals such as potassium and sodium that are extinguished by covering with D̲irt produce type D̲ fires.

Many times fire may be caused by one type of fuel and spread to other fuel types. Most vessels have the potential for types A, B, and C fires. It is unlikely that a dive boat will need to worry about a type D fire. All modern fire extinguishers are clearly labeled for the type of fires they are designed to extinguish. Most fire extinguishers marketed for marine use should be applicable for types A, B, and C fires, but this should be checked before purchase. Fire extinguishers should be inspected yearly and checked for proper pressures monthly.

Type A - Wood or Cloth

The concept in fighting a type A fire is to eliminate unburned fuel from contact with the flame and to **cool the burning fuel**. Simply extinguishing the flame will not stop the fire. If the fuel remains hot (above the ignition temperature of the specific fuel) it will simply reignite and continue burning. The fuel is cooled with large quantities of water doused at the base of the fire (See Figure 72 for Type A Fire). Potential fuel that is in contact with the flame must be cooled as well, such as walls and ceiling areas above the flames. Hidden fire or smoldering fuel can be found behind walls, under floors, above ceilings, and inside containers. All these areas must be exposed and cooled before a fire is considered extinguished.

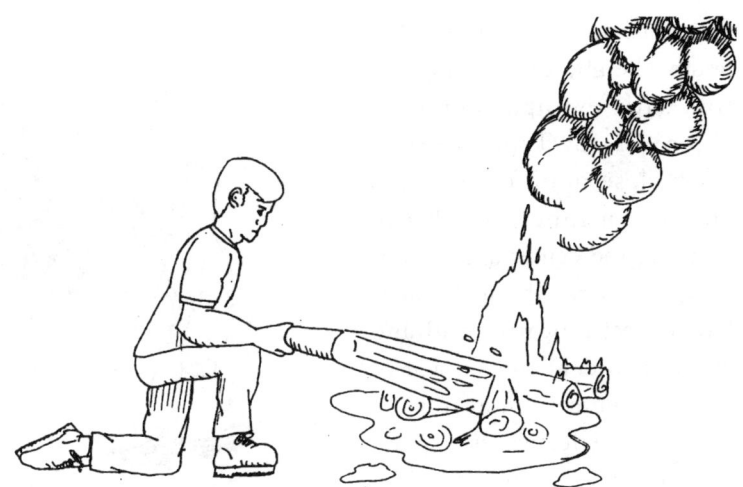

Figure 72 Cooling the fuel of Type A fire by spraying water directly on the base of the fire.

Type B – Liquids

The concept behind extinguishing type B fires is to **separate the flame from the fuel**. Covering the fuel (liquid) with a foam or chemical will accomplish this. Spraying water on liquid fuel will spread the fuel and worsen the problem. Most liquid fuels are lighter than water and will layer out on the surface and continue to burn. The source of the fuel must be stopped. This may be accomplished by closing a gasoline valve, or by removing any other potential sources of fuel (i.e., containers of flammable liquids). These fires also produce large amounts of flammable vapors that can cause explosions.

The extinguishing agents used for type B fires are water fog, dry chemical (i.e., sodium bicarbonate, monoammonium phosphates), chemical foam (i.e., carbon dioxide), mechanical foam (i.e., protein, alcohol, synthetic, or aqueous), and carbon dioxide. The best manner to attack these fires is to first spray the extinguishing agent around the liquid, thereby surrounding the fire with extinguisher (See Figure 73 for Type B Fires). Then close in on the fire in a circular manner, gradually reaching the center and smothering the fire. If the foam is banked off a nearby wall and allowed to coat the surface of the fire, these foam agents are much more effective than spraying directly on the fire (See Figure 74 for banking foam off wall). Rinsing the area with a detergent after the fire is extinguished will help eliminate the fuel and residue from the area.

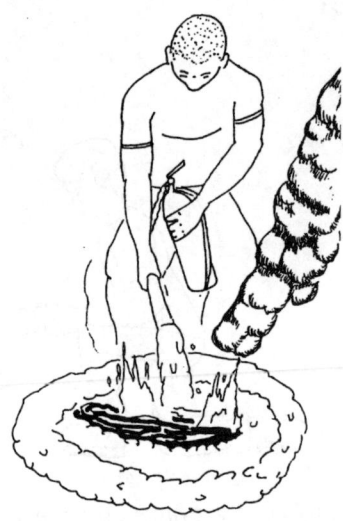

Figure 73 Extinguishing Type B fire by encircling the liquid fuel with foam, then spiraling toward the center.

Type C – Electrical

An arch of current almost always causes electrical fires from an exposed wire or a short from direct contact with a conductive material. The basic concept in extinguishing these fires is to **stop the current**. Shutting off the generator or the fuse will usually accomplish this. It is quite common for electrical fires to spark type A or type B fires. Considerable heat is generated in a very short period of time and other fuels may need to be cooled after the current has been eliminated. A nonconducting agent is best for extinguishing these fires, such as carbon dioxide, dry chemical, or Halon.

Type D – Metals

Flammable metals can be extinguished only by **drying the fuel**. Exposure to water is what produces the chemical reaction

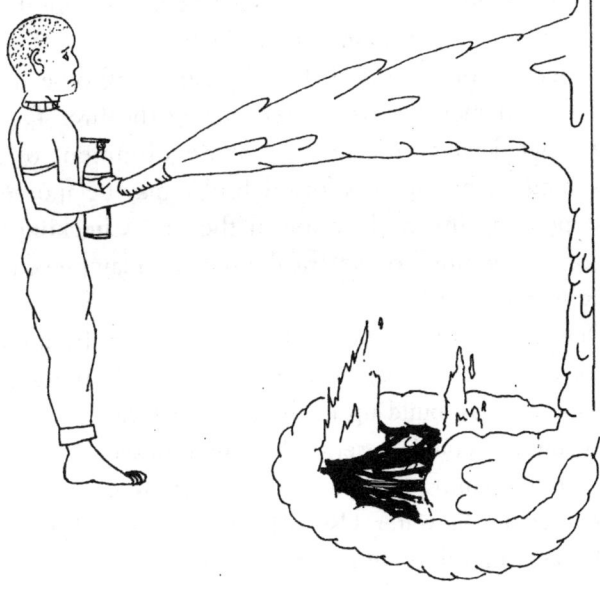

Figure 74 First encircle liquid fuel with foam, then spraying foam at a nearby wall will allow foam to blanket over liquid fuel as it flows down. This avoids dispersing flame by spraying directly at the fire.

that results in the release of energy in the form of flames. Smother the fire with a drying agent such as dirt, sand, or an appropriate extinguisher.

Vessel Inspection and Dewatering

After a fire has been extinguished, the vessel must be inspected for potential smoldering within the wood or fibers. The cabin and bilge must be examined for extension of flames or smoldering beneath or above floors and ceilings. Analysis of the cause of the fire will help prevent recurrence of the problem, whether type A, B, C, or D. If the fire was type C or began as a type C, the electrical power should not be restarted. The power to the engines may be turned on to get back to harbor if that circuit was not the one responsible for the fire.

Inspection of the vessel should include any other potential problem that may have occurred during the fire. These may include weakening of the hull or development of a leak. Weakening of the supports for the bridge may be another problem depending on the location of the fire. Checking for fuel leaks or deterioration of electrical insulation may prevent another emergency.

Dewatering is the process of removing water from the vessel interior after the fire has been extinguished. At times a significant volume may build up in the bilge or other compartments. Vessel stability could be seriously compromised. Automatic and manual bilge pumps, buckets, and other strategies may be needed to evacuate the water. Use as little water as is absolutely necessary to extinguish the fire and cool the fuel.

Vessel Aground

Knowing the draft of the vessel (depth of the hull in the water) and having an accurate depth gauge is important to ensure safe navigability. But there is no substitute for familiarity with the local waterways and a full set of charts to avoid going aground with a boat. Understanding and following day markers is an essential part of remaining within a safe channel.

If a vessel does go aground, the captain will need to assess the damage to the hull and determine whether the vessel is still sea worthy or if the vessel may be taking on water. The safety of the passengers – not the integrity of the vessel – is the number one priority. Surge, current, and waves may be complicating factors and need to be considered when determining the captain's next move. Donning life jackets, the deployment of the life raft, or just jumping off the boat and swimming or walking to shore may be acceptable options.

If there is no leak and other vessels are in the vicinity, they will be in the best position to give assistance with a tow. Calling for help is the next best option but will require a longer time interval before being able to be freed. Time is of the essence more often than not to prevent further damage to the vessel from surge, current, or waves. The tidal effects may be another factor to consider. If the tide is going out, time is much more crucial for getting the vessel out since the problem will get worse as the hull bears a greater proportion of the vessel's weight. If the tide is coming in, time may improve the situation by adding depth to the water, although current may become a factor that may push the vessel toward shallower waters. Placing the anchor out may keep the vessel from moving toward shallower waters as the tide moves in and may allow for the vessel to be freed as the tide raises the vessel.

If the bow is the only part of the hull aground, the captain may attempt to reverse the propellers and pull free. Asking all passengers to move to the rear of the boat to help raise the bow may be of assistance in freeing the boat. Having crew members stand in front of the bow and lift may be of benefit as well (See Figure 75 for lifting bow to free vessel). If the stern (rear) of the vessel has gone aground, do not use the propellers as they

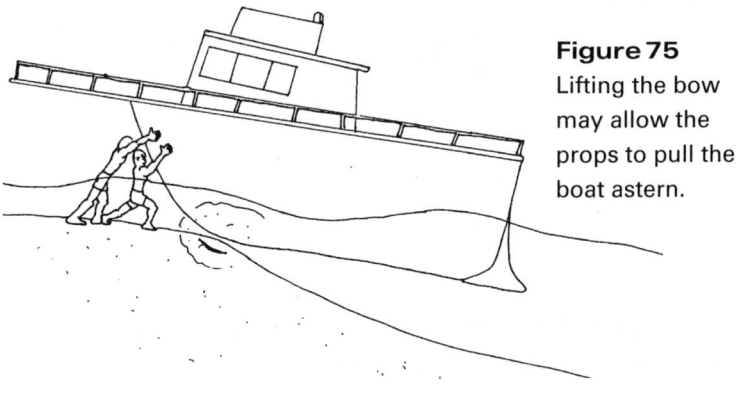

Figure 75
Lifting the bow may allow the props to pull the boat astern.

will be damaged. Instead, the captain can try to either throw or take the anchor in a raft (if the water is shallow enough the anchor could be carried) as far out from shore as possible and attempt to ensure the best purchase (hold of the anchor) as possible. Then ask the passengers to move to the front of the boat to raise the stern and activate the anchor wench. The pull on the anchor may be sufficiently strong to drag the vessel back to deeper water (See Figure 76 for pulling free with anchor). Crew members may also attempt to lift the stern while the anchor wench is pulling the vessel out.

If carrying a heavy load onboard, the captain may decide whether it is worthwhile moving the load forward or back to redistribute the weight or to dump the cargo off the vessel altogether to help raise the hull (See Figure 77 for shifting cargo to free vessel). The cargo can be carried to shore or placed in a raft and then reloaded after the vessel has been freed. Rafts do have a limited capacity for weight and this must be taken into consideration at the time.

Depending on the circumstances there may be other strategies for freeing the vessel but calling the Coast Guard or other assistance by radio or phone soon after going aground is recommended. Harbors, marinas, Coast Guard, conservation police, and bypassing vessels are a few options or organizations that can offer help. Channels 12 and 16 are radio frequencies that are monitored by the EMS.

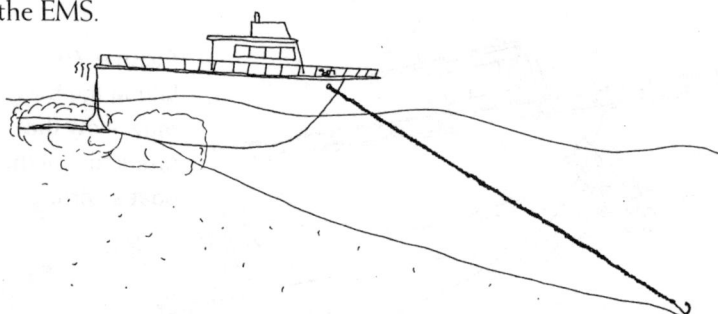

Figure 76 Setting anchor and using the anchor wench to pull a vessel aground out into deeper water.

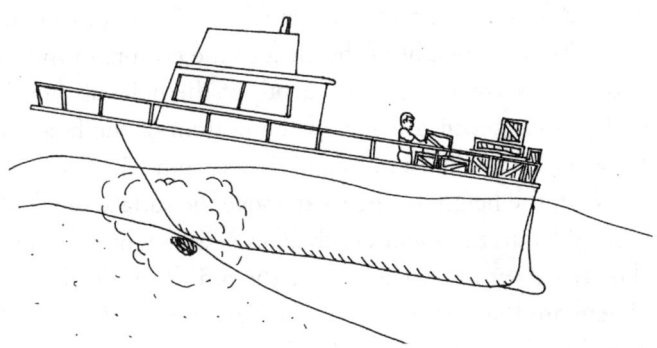

Figure 77 Shifting cargo to the stern may lift the bow and allow the props to pull the boat astern.

Dragging Anchor

Dragging anchor is a fairly common occurrence depending on the bottom composition. The closer one is to shore or other objects, the more significant the implications may be if one is dragging anchor. Having the appropriate size and type of anchor will be essential to prevent this occurrence depending on the size of the vessel and the specific bottom composition. During strong wind, heavy seas, strong current, or significant surge one may consider the use of a second anchor. The second anchor is placed so that the two anchor lines form a "V" shape with an angle from 15 to 45 degrees.

The rode (amount of anchor line let out) will determine the angle of the anchor line and therefore the vertical angle of pull on the anchor. It is recommended that a ration (also known as the scope) of seven to one be used when determining how much length of line to let out in relation to the depth of the water. That is to say, you let out seven feet (or meters) of line for every one foot (or meters) of depth. In strong winds or current, that ratio may be increased to ten to one in order to increase the purchase of the anchor. The "depth" needs to be accurately determined for optimizing anchor purchase. The depth should be measured from the height of the cleat to the bottom of the water. Most operators know the draft (depth of the hull) of their boat. Most depth gauges measure from the bottom of the boat to the sea floor. These two must be added to determine the depth of the water. Next, the height of the cleat above the surface of the water must be added to the water depth. This final height is then multiplied by seven (or ten) to determine the rode of the anchor.

There are four main methods of determining if one is dragging anchor. The easiest, most high-tech method is the use of the GPS. The GPS will let one know one's position within several feet and a constantly changing bearing will confirm drift by the boat. Many GPS units have an anchor drag setting that will sound an alarm if the boat moves a preprogrammed specified distance. One may need to choose the preprogrammed distance wisely to avoid the GPS from alarming if the boat swings around the anchor due to wind direction changes.

Fixing your position on visual landmarks bases another method of determining anchor drag (See Figure 78 for using landmarks to check for anchor drag). This method of determining one's position is based on the premise that one is close to land. The closer one is to land the more accurate one can be

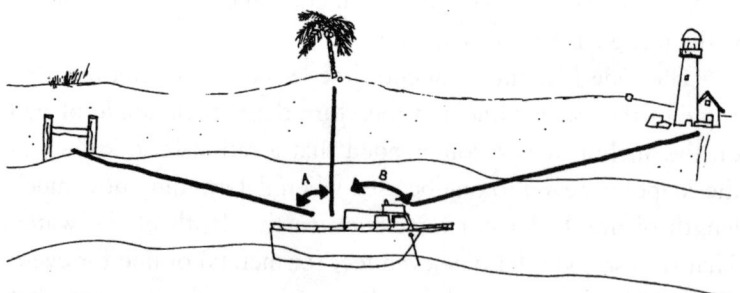

Figure 78 Obtain bearings on several fixed objects and plot the angle between them.

about the vessel's stationary position. Always use fixed objects or landmarks, not floating, anchored, or moored objects. One should take a bearing (compass setting) on at least two stationary objects and plot the angle between the two and the vessel. Three or four objects can be used and will make the position more accurate. For increased accuracy one should choose landmarks whose lines of direction from the boat intersect at angles near 90 degrees. Three bearings that intersect at angles of about 60 degrees give one a better position. Any drift of the vessel will change the angle formed by the lines plotted from the landmarks to the boat. This method requires much more vigilance by the captain (See Figure 79 for angle change of landmarks during anchor drag). A significantly greater distance of drag may occur before drag is suspected or confirmed than with GPS.

The third method of establishing anchor drag is by fixing the position of the vessel using radar ranges. Radar can be used to determine accurate distances and direction of landmarks and stationary objects even in reduced visibility. Because of the way radar works it is able to determine distances much more accurately than direction and therefore distance rather than direction is routinely used to determine anchor drag. Using a ruler or a plotting

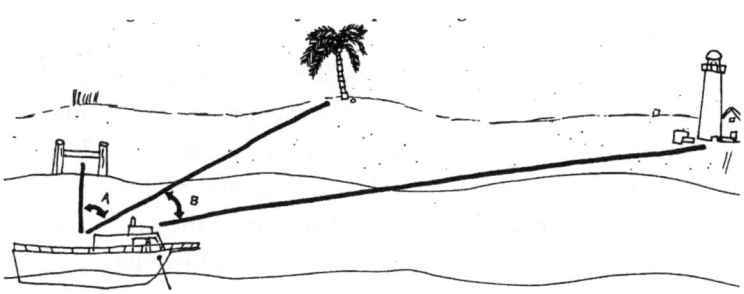

Figure 79 Anchor drag can be established if the angle between the bearings of the objects change.

compass, one can measure distances from objects picked up by the radar screen and monitor those distances for change (See Figure 80 for radar ranges to monitor anchor drag). One can plot the position on a chart if desired but simply monitoring the distances on the screen should suffice to check for anchor drag.

Figure 80 A change in the distance of objects on radar will detect anchor drag.

The fourth method of determining anchor drag is with the use of a drift lead. This is a useful method if there is poor visibility, no landmarks, or no GPS is available. One ties a lead weight to a line and drops it to the sea floor. Pay out enough slack to allow for swings of the vessel on the anchor line and tie the line to a cleat or rail. If the line becomes taut and pulls parallel to the anchor line one is dragging anchor (See Figure 81 to check for anchor drag with drift load).

If dragging anchor has been established, one can weigh (lift) the anchor and attempt to re-cast the anchor to achieve a better location for anchor purchase. Paying out more rode may improve the anchor's purchase. Use of a second anchor may also help eliminate drag. Divers may also inspect the anchor when descending to ensure no drag is occurring before they venture off to their dive destination.

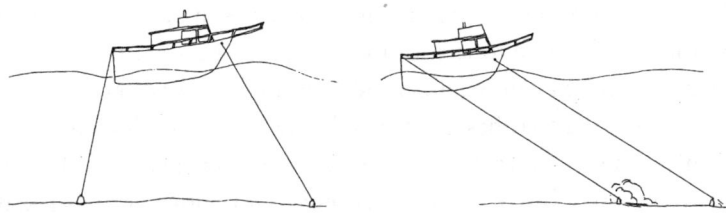

Figure 81 Anchor drag is established if the line of the drift lead becomes parallel to the anchor line.

Power Failure

Engine Failure

Engine failure may be the result of being out of fuel, mechanical problems, or propeller damage. Maintaining a full fuel tank, proper engine maintenance, and vigilance to water depth can preclude the vast majority of preventable causes of engine failure. Constant attention to fuel and oil levels during a cruise will alert the vessel operator of fuel or oil consumption or leaks. Always check the oil before departing on an excursion. Except for fuel problems, a vessel with two or more engines will make the return to port possible, albeit slower and more challenging if one engine malfunctions. If propeller damage is the cause of engine failure, preventing propeller damage to the second engine is paramount. If shallow water was the cause of propeller damage to one engine, getting a tow from another vessel or using the anchor to pull the vessel into deeper water may protect the second propeller in a twin engine vessel.

Another difficult problem may be removing twine or rope that has been wrapped around the propeller blade. Having a diver go under the vessel to cut or untangle the material from the propeller could be dangerous, especially in rough water.

Conducting an engine repair in open water may be difficult if not impossible due to lack of tools or parts. Most of the time an engine problem will require a tow in a single engine vessel.

An engine that has overheated may be the result of running it at too high of a throttle, a closed water intake valve, a broken water pump, a broken or plugged hose, or debris getting sucked into the cooling system intake. If a piece of plastic or other debris is stuck on the water intake, a brief snorkel under the vessel may find and correct the problem. Care is needed when swimming under the boat in rough water. At times the intake valve may have been shut off during repairs or maintenance and simply needs to be re-opened. If overheating was due to running the engine too high, shutting down the engine for a time will cool the engine. Then restarting the engine and running it at lower rpm's may resolve the problem. If the engine continues to overheat, it is likely due to one of the other reasons and may be shut down in order to return to harbor with one engine. An engine that is overheating and shut off can be used intermittently at crucial periods for better maneuverability such as when needed for mooring, if in proximity to obstacles or land, or near other vessels. One may run a low risk of engine damage but this possibility may need to be balanced against the risk of injury or vessel damage.

Some of the most dangerous situations confronted during engine failure have to do with rough seas when close to shore. If the vessel is close to shore or other obstructions the judicious use of an anchor is advised. Use a second anchor if there is doubt about the purchase of the anchor. Calling for help is mandatory.

Electrical Failure

Lack of fuel may also be a cause of concomitant power failure due to a loss of generator function. Battery function may be spared but if also affected, calling for help may be facilitated with a battery-operated, hand-held ship to shore radio or portable phone. In the case of a complete electrical failure, vital systems such as electric bilge pumps, depth gauges, fuel and oil gauges, GPS, Loran, lights, and sensors will all be inactivated. In these circumstances the vessel operators will need to be more vigilant than usual to their location, course, and engine function.

At times the problem is not fuel, but rather that the generator battery is discharged and the generator won't crank to start. On most vessels the generator and the engines have separate batteries. These may be interposed if one is discharged and the other is still charged.

Bad Weather and Rough Water

Bad weather and rough water usually go hand in hand and develop at the same time. Wind speed is one of the determinants of wave height along with water depth and the fetch (distance that the wind has to blow over and influence the water). The direction of the current will also have an influence on the peaking of the waves depending on the direction of the wind. Wind that blows over water that has a current in the opposite direction will have waves that are more peaked, thus causing a rougher cruise. Rain, hale, lightning, wind, and microbursts may all be compounding problems that a vessel may have to deal with during a storm.

The best protection from bad or changing weather is constant monitoring of the weather channel on the ship to shore radio or an AM/FM radio. Listening to the weather forecast the day before a dive will alert the diver or the vessel operator of the potential for poor weather conditions. The forecast is usually more accurate the morning of the dive. Most harbors will display small craft and storm warnings. It would be wise to take notice of these warnings before starting out on a cruise. **If in doubt, don't go out!** It is best to err on the side of caution and dive another day rather than to brave a risky day that may end in tragedy.

Understanding weather patterns and keeping a watchful eye on the skies may alert a captain or vessel operator of an approaching front. Anvil-shaped or dark and billowing clouds (cumulo-nimbus clouds), a sudden change in the air temperature, wind direction, and wind speed are common warning signs of approaching storms. Lightning in the distance is an ominous sign of trouble. Weather fronts frequently approach with incredible speed and can turn a calm setting into a nightmare within a very short time span. High altitude feathery clouds (cirrus clouds) often are warning signs of worsening weather. The white and puffy low altitude clouds (cumulus clouds) are indicative of continued fair weather in the area.

If there are divers in the water and any sign of changing weather conditions are visible or an alert is heard on the radio, the captain should sound the call back signal immediately. It may take a significant period of time to round up all the divers and get them all onboard the vessel. All gear that can be brought to the interior should be stowed away in an expeditious manner and secured. All tanks need to be properly secured on deck. All hatches and windows should be closed and anchor should be weighed (raised). A head count is mandatory before leaving the area.

The most direct heading toward safe harbor should be initiated at the most rapid speed the captain may determine to be safe. The vessel should head toward the closest harbor even if not the home harbor. If the vessel is between harbors, a heading toward the harbor furthest away from the approaching storm front should be made. This will give the vessel more time to get to safe harbor before the storm arrives. A heading into the approaching front may be ill advised.

If rough weather or water conditions are encountered, the captain or vessel operator should first have all crew and passengers don their life vests. Passengers should remain inside the cabin if there is one, or at least stay away from the sides or railings of the vessel to prevent a man overboard scenario. Hatches and windows are closed to prevent taking on water. All gear is either brought inside the cabin or properly secured.

Taking a tack that takes the waves on an angle is usually the best course. Keeping the vessel from taking a wave broadside is usually recommended to reduce the likelihood of capsizing. The velocity of the vessel will need to be adjusted to keep the vessel's bow from submarining when the waves are coming from the bow. Likewise, if the waves are approaching from the stern, the velocity of the vessel may be adjusted to prevent the waves from washing over the transom and flooding the vessel.

If the vessel capsizes, passengers within the cabin may attempt to exit the cabin before it completely fills with water. This may be nearly impossible from the force of the water pouring in through the hatches, windows, or entrance. At times, the easiest method to exit may be to allow the cabin to flood and then swim out after the water movement through the opening has slowed down. Waiting for the vessel to fill with water may be difficult from a psychological standpoint but may be the only means of exit. The victims of a capsized vessel should attempt to hold onto a rigid object near the point of exit as the vessel fills with water to stay in proximity to the point of exit. This will facilitate finding the point of exit in the dark, under water once the vessel's cabin has flooded and exit is possible. The victims need to take care to avoid entanglement within the cabin or being caught within an opening or hatch that is too small to allow exit. A victim with a life vest on may need to swim to a deeper point within the cabin to reach the exit. They will need to remove and abandon their flotation vest as it will push them upward and not allow them to dive down to reach the exit of a capsized vessel.

Many vessels are designed to stay at the surface despite being flooded and capsized. Victims of a capsized vessel should stay clear of the vessel but remain in its proximity. If the vessel remains at the surface, attempts should be made to climb onto the capsized vessel. This would make finding the victim much easier during a rescue since the vessel would be a much more sightable object than a lone swimmer in the water. In addition, the victim would reduce the likelihood of hypothermia by staying out of the water as much as possible. Other benefits of remaining on the capsized vessel would include being able to keep a group together, prevention of injury from marine predators, avoidance of fatigue, and having access to potential provisions that may still be within the flooded cabin.

CHAPTER SEVEN

Travel-Related Conditions

A traveler needs to assume an air of confidence and at the same time maintain a sense of healthy paranoia while traveling abroad. Dangers and risks are everywhere in the world from a variety of sources. A foreigner in a strange land is vulnerable to disease, villains, and shysters. Care must be taken to avoid disease or assault while traveling.

If in a foreign country and a crisis or emergency occurs, the Bureau of Consular Affairs can be a great resource to coordinate assistance. The bureau may issue a passport in case of loss or theft. In case of an emergency at home, the bureau can help locate and notify the traveling party of the problem. In case of injury or illness, the bureau can help find medical or dental help, coordinate a task force to notify family, assist in transfer of funds, obtain medical records of the injured American to the treating physician, and arrange in transporting the injured American back to the United States. All funds and costs are the responsibility of the victim or their family but the time and effort to coordinate services will be assumed by the Bureau of Consular Affairs.

In case of a natural disaster or political upheaval, the Bureau of Consular Affairs can coordinate a task force to evacuate Americans.

If commercial transportation is interrupted, the bureau can arrange or charter special transportation through Washington to bring Americans to the United States or to safety. If you are arrested the consular can assist you and your family with services. In case of a death of an American in a foreign country, the bureau will locate and inform the next of kin. The bureau will assist the family in arrangements for burial or return of the remains to the United States. A Foreign Service Report of Death will be prepared by the consular officer based on the local death certificate and supply it to the next of kin.

Contacting the embassy and/or the travel ministries of the intended destinations may alert the traveler to epidemics, pandemics, social or political upheaval, required vaccines, and recommended medication. Libraries, newspapers, and the Internet are other sources of local news and advisories of the intended destination.

Air Travel

Air travel poses several risks to travelers that range from illness to injury. Exposure to burglary has also been described in a variety of ways. The astute and seasoned traveler will take precautions to avoid or at least minimize exposure.

Burglary

Keeping bags close at hand and never putting your laptop, briefcase, or purse on the floor will lessen the risk of being robbed at an airport. Once the luggage has been checked in, it is out of your control and at the mercy of bag handlers. It has been reported on several occasions that bag handlers are notorious for possessing a collection of keys to open just about any bag lock that requires a key. They have been videotaped searching through passengers' bags in a variety of areas in an airport. The best advice is to use a high quality combination lock. Wrapping or taping a bag further deters searching through bags. Many times the entire bag is stolen and listed as "lost." It is not uncommon to have a bag end up in a different destination than the passenger. Airlines will limit reimbursement of lost items to a nominal fee. They will pay for damage up to a minimal amount.

When passing through the airport, it is recommended to have covered suitcase address tags to prevent advertising your address. It may be a good idea to substitute your office or work address for that of your home. Crafty burglars will know you are out of town and take note of your home address. Especially when traveling with the whole family, beware of friendly ticket agents or fellow passengers. Recent reports of a burglary ring were discovered where the ticket agent was the "brains" of the operation taking the address, dates of departure and return, and making friendly conversation with passengers to find out if the whole family was traveling. The homes of their victims were then robbed during their trip.

Conditions Encountered in Flight
•Decompression Illness

Divers on the return flight from a dive trip need to be most concerned about decompression illness. It is most widely recommended that divers wait 24 hours after a no-decompression dive. If a decompression dive was performed, a 48-hour wait is recommended. Even using these parameters air passengers have suffered from the bends after diving. If a diver begins to experience symptoms of decompression illness (see section on decompression illness for a list of possible symptoms) the victim should be laid down and given oxygen.

The flight attendant should be notified immediately and the pilot appraised of the situation. If the pressure within the cabin can be increased it should be done as quickly as possible. The altitude of the flight should be taken down to the lowest allowable altitude and the closest airport must be identified where a decompression chamber is located to make an emergency landing to de-plane the victim. If the pilot calls ahead an ambulance will be waiting to transport the victim to the hyperbaric chamber. Calling ahead will prepare the chamber for the victim in order to expedite treatment.

•Deep Vein Thrombosis and Pulmonary Embolus

In prolonged flights where the passengers are sitting for multiple hours, a silent and deadly condition can sneak up on a traveler. The circulation in the legs slows to dangerously low velocities and the blood tends to pool in the distended veins in the legs. This stagnated blood increases its coagulability (ability to form clots) and clots begin to form in the veins in the calf, behind the knee, or deep in the thighs (deep vein thrombosis). These clots in the leg veins may dislodge and embolize to the lungs (pulmonary embolus) where they occlude the circulation of blood flowing through the lungs. Small clots may be tolerated and may even go unnoticed but large clots will significantly affect circulation and oxygenation of blood and can quickly lead to death. Walking, contracting the leg muscles, or massaging the calves may dislodge the thrombus from the leg.

The signs of a deep vein thrombosis are swelling of the legs. It is especially suspicious if only one foot or leg is swollen. Pain in the calf or behind the knees is the most common complaint. Victims often have tenderness of the calf upon flexing the ankle upward, squeezing the calf, or pushing on the area behind the knee. Feeling a "cord" in the calf or behind the knee is frequently encountered on examination. Care is taken to not dislodge a thrombus (clot) while examining the victim. The exam is done gently with a soft touch. Symptoms include pain, numbness, or discomfort of the foot or calf or a sense of heaviness in the leg. When a pulmonary embolus occurs the victim may have no symptoms if the embolus is small, or they may die immediately if a massive thrombus embolizes. If a moderate-sized embolus occurs the victim may experience shortness of breath, chest pain, and palpitations. If an embolus occurs, recurrent emboli could follow in short order and may increase in size. Deep vein thrombosis and pulmonary embolus are extreme medical emergencies.

Prevention of deep vein thrombosis is by exercising the leg muscles frequently while sitting. Getting up and walking around the cabin of the plane is recommended a few times an hour. Taking an aspirin before a long flight may decrease the coagulability of the blood and may reduce the risk of a deep vein thrombosis. If a thrombosis is suspected the goal is to prevent it from embolizing to the lungs. Elevation of the affected leg and immobilizing it are important. Avoid massaging or milking the leg. Do not exercise the leg muscles and avoid walking. Immediate medical attention is mandatory.

If a pulmonary embolus is suspected and the victim has survived, prevention of further emboli is paramount by the above recommendations. High concentrations of oxygen are given to the victim until they are taken to a medical facility.

•Respiratory Infections

It has been well documented that respiratory infections spread within the confined cabins of an airplane. Influenza, cold viruses, and tuberculosis are amongst the most worrisome infections because of their contagiousness from airborne particles. Infectious droplets from a cough or sneeze can travel several feet and may be aided by the flow of ventilation within the plane's cabin.

If one is assigned a seat near or next to a coughing passenger, one should cover one's mouth and nose with a filter such as a tissue for several seconds after they cough. Avoid handling or touching objects that the ill passenger has handled after they have covered their mouth while coughing. Do not allow the ill passenger to pass food or drink from the flight attendant to you. One may direct the air vent so the flow will direct the air away from oneself. One may request being seated far away from the ill passenger, especially behind the ill passenger if possible.

•Turbulence

Turbulence during flight is a common encounter and can produce anxiety or injury. Individuals already apprehensive about flying can become even more anxious and could even precipitate a panic attack. The judicial use of anti-anxiety medications taken before flying may have a beneficial effect to help calm the nervous passenger.

Severe turbulence could cause the plane to tilt or to lose altitude unexpectedly. These disturbances in smooth flight could cause articles to be flung through the cabin causing significant injury to passengers. Passengers who are not strapped into their seat belts or who are walking or standing in the cabin could be tossed into other passengers or caused to strike the ceiling, walls, or seats within the cabin with tremendous force and cause a variety of serious injuries. Hot beverages or food could be spilled onto passengers and cause injuries or discomfort.

It is recommended that all articles be stowed away in the overhead compartments or under the seat in front of the passenger to avoid having them become projectiles during such an event. These overhead compartments need to be opened cautiously after a flight to be sure they have not shifted during the flight, causing them to fall out and injure someone when the compartments are opened. It is recommended that all passengers wear their seat belts in a snug manner to prevent or minimize injury during severe turbulence.

Should an injury occur during a period of severe turbulence, it is recommended that the victim be placed in their seat and their seat belt applied to prevent further injury should turbulence continue to occur. The individual who is to evaluate them should sit beside them with their seat belt on to avoid injury themselves if the problem does recur. It may be appropriate to ask if there is a physician on board who could evaluate and direct treatment to the victim. Flight attendants do receive training for first aid and in-flight injuries and they may be the best individuals to coordinate assistance. All planes are equipped with a first aid kit for treatment of minor injuries.

If the victim has lost consciousness or is dazed they should have multiple blankets placed around them to pad the window and to attempt to stabilize them within their seat. Placing a blanket around the victim and tying it around the seat back or having the person sitting behind them hold the blanket ends may help keep the victim from flinging around in their seat during further turbulence (See Figure 82 for restraining victim during turbulence). Rolling up a blanket lengthwise and gently wrapping it around the victim's head and neck may reduce whiplash and stabilize the cervical spine. An evaluation of the possible

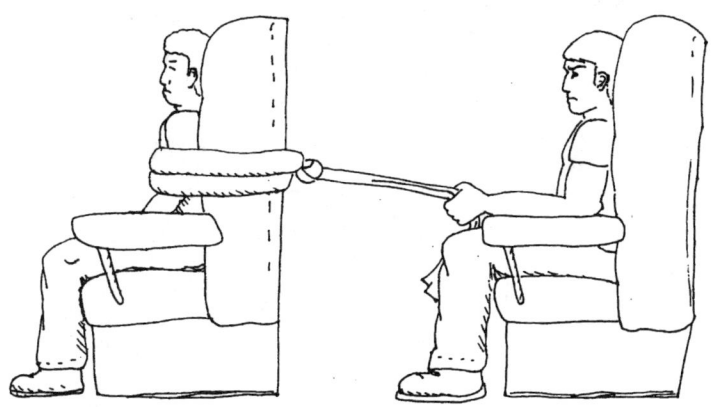

Figure 82 Stabilizing a dazed or unconscious victim in their seat during severe turbulence.

injuries and the appropriate treatment should be instituted to stabilize their injuries and prevent further injury.

If a spine injury is suspected, the victim may be placed flat on the floor in the aisle (See Figure 83 for securing spine victim during turbulence). Blankets may be used to strap the victim to the floor in case of further turbulence. The blankets may be placed around the seat legs on either side of the victim. The passengers in the seats just behind these seats may hold the blanket ends and place a foot on the blanket to the side of the victim to hold them down. Blankets may be placed across the chest, pelvis, knees, or feet to secure the victim to the floor. The head may be secured by holding or being wedged with cloth on either side. If serious injury is suspected and emergency medical attention is required, the pilot should be notified in order to find the nearest landing site to expedite definitive medical treatment to the victim.

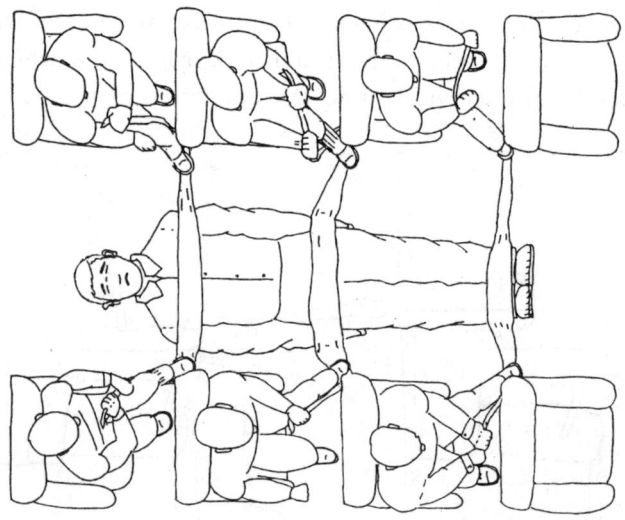

Figure 83 Securing a suspected spine injury victim to the floor during turbulence.

•Jet Lag

Jet lag, otherwise known as desynchronosis, is a condition that affects travelers when they travel across several time zones within a short period of time. The severity of the symptoms may vary depending on the individual, the length of travel time, and the number of time zones crossed. The problem arises when the internal clock that controls day/night cycles (circadian rhythms) is out of sync with the environment and one's activities. This disorder of wakefulness and sleep usually lasts only a few days and may vary depending on the individual's activities and the number of time zones off-sync one is. Travelers may experience similar or even more severe symptoms upon returning to their original time zone after their trip.

The most common symptoms are those of insomnia (inability to sleep) at night and sleepiness or fatigue during daytime hours. Travelers may experience swings in their level of alertness during the first few days. Other symptoms frequently encountered during jet lag are decreased concentration and alertness, headaches, abdominal pain, irritability, and dizziness.

Early morning travelers who are westbound (up to a certain distance) may find it easier to accommodate since it has been found that extending one's day and staying awake longer is easier to adjust to than traveling eastbound the same distance where the traveler would be shortening their day. Eastbound travelers may elect to travel late at night and arrive during the day at their destination to once again attempt to prolong their day rather than attempt to shorten their waking time period.

If traveling across more than six time zones, one may elect to adjust one's sleeping period during the trip to ready one's system for the time one is to arrive. For instance, if one will be arriving in the morning at their destination site they may try to sleep as much as possible during travel so that one's system is rested once they arrive in order to stay up that day. Conversely, if one were to arrive at night at the destination site, one would try to stay awake during the trip so that their body is tired and can sleep once they arrive. These strategies may help but it will still take a few days to adjust one's internal cycles. The traveler may also consider adjusting their sleep patterns gradually over several days prior to departure if their schedules allow in an attempt to simulate their intended time zone.

A traveler who is already well rested prior to departure will find that they can make the adjustment easier. The use of caffeine at the beginning of the new day period may help a recent traveler stay awake, but the "let-down" after the caffeine has worn off may be much more intense. Avoiding caffeine later in the day may allow the traveler to sleep easier the first few nights. Short acting hypnotics (sleeping pills) may be of benefit the first few nights. Exposure to bright light during the morning and early afternoon and dimmed lighting in the late afternoon and evening can hasten adjustment to the new time zone. Some travelers claim that the use of melatonin, a neurotransmitter produced in the pineal gland of the brain that helps regulate the circadian rhythm, is helpful in the treatment of jet lag. Its efficacy has not been proven.

The traveling scuba diver may want to take into consideration knowledge of how jet lag may affect their concentration and energy level to plan their dive schedules. The diver may elect to not dive for the first few days until their circadian rhythms have accommodated to the new time zone. Alternatively they may try to schedule their first few days of diving during times that their waking periods at both time zones would overlap.

Parasites

There are many types of parasites. Many are external and live on the skin of the host, either temporarily (i.e., mosquito) or permanently (i.e., tick or mite). Other parasites are internal and reside within the intestine or internal organs. These parasites may gain access to the host by being ingested or by penetrating the skin. Divers who are traveling may be at risk for several reasons. Residing in transient living quarters, often in remote and underdeveloped areas, exposing their skin due to the nature of their sport, and often eating exotic meals from facilities that may have sub-optimal quality and inspection standards make divers susceptible to parasites.

An organism may be considered a parasite if it lives on or within another organism (a host) and depends upon the host for protection, nutrition, or transportation. Some of these parasite/host relationships may be mutually beneficial to both the parasite and the host; this is known as a symbiotic or mutualistic relationship. If one (the parasite) is the only one receiving the benefit and the host is neither benefiting nor being hurt, the relationship between the two is known as commensalism. Parasitism is a term usually reserved for a relationship where the parasite is receiving all the benefit and inflicts some degree of injury or damage on the host. Most animals in nature have hundreds or millions of parasites. In fact, the majority of parasites act as hosts to other smaller parasites in nature.

Parasites are one of the most successful organisms on the planet. Their numbers and their ability to find and infest their hosts are incredible. Humans are universally used as hosts to some parasites, and most people have multiple species. Travelers may become hosts to parasites when their guard is let down in foreign counties or rural areas where proper hygiene and sanitary conditions are less than optimal. Individuals who travel can forget that the health standards may be significantly lower than what they are used to. Being naive to the risks of parasitic infestation is a main reason travelers fall prey to these opportunistic organisms. It is important to know how these parasites are transmitted to be able to take the proper precautions to avoid exposure.

Class Insecta

The parasites of the class Insecta are comprised of a collection of insects that are external parasites. Most of these feed off the blood of the host while some lay their eggs beneath the skin. Although these insects are for the most part bothersome and in themselves cause minimal injury, it is the diseases they can transmit to the host that possess the major health risk.

Prevention of becoming the host is the best management. Staying out of the brush in remote areas, keeping one's distance from animals, and the use of a potent insect repellent are key strategies of avoidance. If entering the brush and wooded areas is necessary, one may consider the use of long pants and sleeves that close tightly around the ankles and wrists.

•Lice (Family Pediculidae)

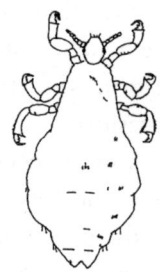

Figure 84 Lice

Lice can carry the virus for swine fever, tularemia and leishmaniasis, rickettsia that causes typhus, cholera, impetigo, trachoma, and the spirochetes that cause trench fever. Lice can be acquired by proximity to others who are infested or by resting in chairs or beds where infested individuals have been. Use of Kwell shampoo or lotion, or Scabene lotion along with repeat shampooing several days later to kill the newly hatched eggs will cure the infestation. (See Figure 84)

•Bedbugs (Family Cimicidae)

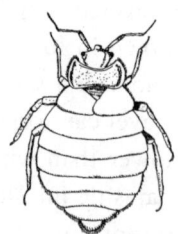

Figure 85 Bedbug

Bedbugs transmit no known diseases but are a major nuisance to travelers. They are known to harbor the hepatitis B virus although transmission to humans has been poorly documented. Cleaning the bed covering and using the appropriate insecticide usually will correct the infestation. One may consider changing accommodations to another resort if bedbugs are a problem. (See Figure 85)

•Fleas (Order Siphonaptera)

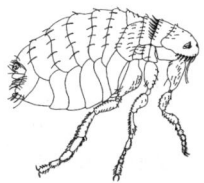

Figure 86 Flea

Fleas carry the organisms that cause Bubonic plague, typhus, tularemia, salmonella, virus of myxomatosis, the cysticercoid stage of several tapeworms, and the larva of the filarial worm. Fleas are usually acquired by proximity to dogs, cats, goats, cattle, or in areas where these animals have been. The nests of fleas may be within linens, rugs, or drapes. An appropriate insecticide will kill the fleas and a repeat treatment after the offspring hatch may be required. Application of an insect repellent will usually do to rid one of fleas. (See Figure 86)

•Sandflies (Family Psychodidae)

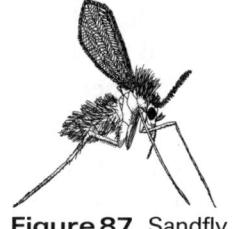

Figure 87 Sandfly

Sandflies can be found in moist, shaded areas during the day and only females suck blood at night. These insects are poor flyers and therefore are usually out on calm, windless evenings.

Sandflies can carry the organism leishmania. Use of an insect repellent is usually effective. Use of long tucked or strapped pants and sleeves is recommended. (See Figure 87)

•Tsetse Fly (Family Muscidae)

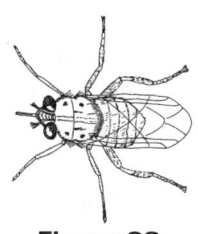

Figure 88
Tsetse Fly

The tsetse fly is a close relative to the common housefly and may carry the organism that is responsible for African sleeping sickness. These bloodsucking flies have a proboscis that contains a bulb at the base of the feeding tube.

Insect repellents are the best precautionary step to preventing their bites. Use of long tucked or strapped pants and sleeves is recommended.(See Figure 88)

• Ticks (Family Ixodidae)

Ticks may carry organisms that can cause Lime disease, borellia, Rocky Mountain fever, tularemia, and Texas cattle fever. Wearing long sleeves and tucking the shirt into the pants and tucking the pants into the socks along with wearing a hat may help protect the individual in a tick-infested location. There are several tick repellents commercially available.

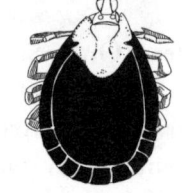

Figure 89 Tick

If a tick is found on the body, simply grasping it by the head with a pair of tweezers and pulling it off may be effective. Acaricides are agents that kill these parasites and they have been evolving since DDT, a once favorite acaricide that has been banned due to its toxicity and cancer-causing potential. There has also been resistance developed by ticks to many of these agents. Suffocation of the ticks has also been advocated. A thick application of olive oil followed by covering the person's head with a plastic cap has been effective for overnight use. Others have advocated applying fingernail polish to the entire tick. Save the tick once removed for analysis for diseases that may have been transmitted to the individual. (See Figure 89)

• Mites (Phylum Arthropoda)

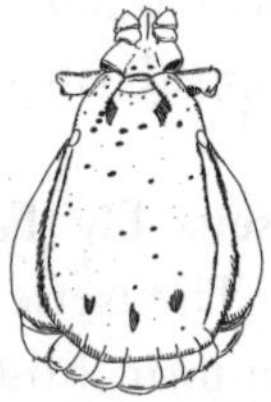

Mites are the smaller cousins of ticks and cause scabies (scab forming, non-burrowing species that live externally) and mange

Figure 90 Mite

(burrowing species that live beneath the skin). Most species are free-living but several species are parasitic and are lymph feeders or bloodsuckers. Most mites live in temperate climates. They can carry the organism that causes typhus. Acaricides are available but again toxicity and resistance may be factors to consider. Kwell cream, Kwell shampoo, and Kwell lotion are known to be effective as well as Scabene lotion. (See Figure 90)

•Mosquitoes (Family Culicidae)

Mosquitoes are the most common pests encountered on dive trips. There are over 2,000 species of mosquitoes and are found worldwide. They are usually just annoying pests but can carry malaria, dengue fever, yellow fever, elephantiasis, flagellates, ciliates, filaria, mites, possibly hepatitis, and midges. The larvae live in water and must surface to get oxygen. Adding oil to water prevents the larva from getting air and kills the larva. Insect repellent is usually effective in preventing bites by the adult mosquito. Use of long pants and sleeves may offer some protection. (See Figure 91)

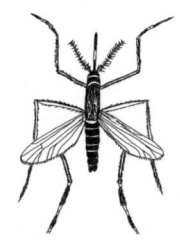

Figure 91
Mosquito

•Blackflies and Buffalo Gnats (Family Simuliidae)

This family of insects has a worldwide distribution. They commonly occur in large swarms and have vicious bites that cause considerable annoyance. The bites cause significant blood loss and the potential for secondary bacterial infection. The saliva is also known to contain toxic chemicals. These insects carry roundworms in Central America, Africa, and Mexico. Tularemia and protozoan parasites are also carried. Insect repellents are usually only partially effective. Long pants and sleeves may help to protect the skin. (See Figure 92)

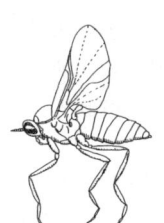

Figure 92
Black Fly

Class Hirudinea

•Leeches

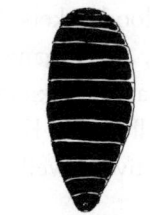

Figure 93 Leech

Leeches belong to this interesting class of organisms. Leeches fall somewhere between parasite and predator since they are known to swallow insect larvae, worms, and snails whole. They can ingest two to five times their weight in blood in a single meal. One species found in Asia, the Middle East, southern Europe, and Africa called *Limnatis nilotica* may be acquired by drinking contaminated water and infest the lungs and upper intestine and cause severe injury to the human host.

Leeches are stimulated to feed by water disturbance. Once attached to the skin, a leech can cut through the skin in less than one minute and begin feeding. Land leeches will climb onto leaves or branches and attach to a bypassing host upon contact. Even small openings of clothing such as the eyelets of boots are enough to let a land leech penetrate one's clothing. It is therefore recommended to wear full-length clothing with tight ankle and wrist ends or tuck ones pants into the socks. Use of insecticides or insect repellents is effective against land leeches.

Simply pulling them off does remove leeches. A strong salt solution has been successful in causing the leeches to detach. Other strategies have been advocated for leeches in the nose and mouth that include the use of lidocaine or cocaine to anesthetize the leech.

Leeches do not transmit any diseases to man. The area where the leech was attached will itch for several days and may be subject to risk of infection and bleeding, at times profusely. The more serious areas of leech attachment may be the eyes, anus, urethra, vagina, and nose. Medical attention should be sought for involvement of these anatomical areas. (See Figure 93)

Class Trematoda

• **Fluke Worms**

These parasites are commonly known as fluke worms. They are known to be endemic in 71 countries. It is estimated that one in twelve people in the world are

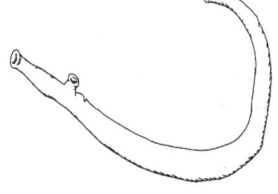

Figure 94 Fluke Worm

infected with a member of this class of parasite. *Schistosoma japonicum*, *Schistosoma haematobium*, and *Schistosoma mansoni* are the three most common species that affect humans. Humans are their definitive host and snails are their intermediate host. Humans may become infected from eating infected snails, although it is known that infection could also occur from direct penetration of the skin by the cercarial stage of the worm while swimming in contaminated water. Flukes can invade the intestinal wall, the lungs, liver, brain, as well as other organs.

Seawater is safe for swimming although rivers, streams, lakes, and the mouths of rivers into the ocean may pose a risk for infection. Chlorinating water and pools will kill the worms. If skin contact with contaminated water occurs, rapid drying or washing with alcohol will prevent infection. If infected or suspected contamination occurs seek medical attention for treatment. Bilticide is an effective anti-schistosomal agent. (See Figure 94)

Class Cestoidea

Parasites in this class of organisms that affect man are the intestinal tapeworms. These parasites have a complex life cycle that consists of an egg stage, a larval stage, then an adult stage. The risk of infestation to humans may be from one or more of the stages of their life cycle. Although the United States and England are amongst the countries with the lowest incidence, these parasites are very common worldwide with a global incidence of two to three percent of the world's population. Mexico, Central America, and the Caribbean have an especially high incidence of these parasites. Asia and Europe have moderately high incidences of these parasites in certain geographical areas.

• **Pork Tapeworm** *(Taenia solium)*

Also known as the pork tapeworm, Taenia solium is a very common parasite in Mexico and Central America where the incidence of human infestation in certain geographical area is as high as eight percent of the population.

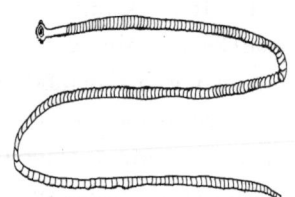

Figure 95 Tape Worm

The adult tapeworm varies in length from six to twenty-one feet (two to seven meters). (See Figure 95) The adult tapeworm releases thousands of eggs that are passed along with the stool of the host. Infested food handlers with poor hygiene may contaminate food with the eggs that are then eaten by others. Food such as salads, vegetables, and fruits that are eaten raw are the most likely culprits to carry the eggs. Individuals that consume the eggs may then become the intermediate host when the eggs hatch and the larva penetrate the intestinal wall and migrate to the host's organs. All organs can become infested with the larval stage known as cysticercosis, commonly including the brain and muscle. It is estimated that in Mexico 60% of all abnormalities seen on brain scans are due to this parasite. The most common intermediate host of this parasite is the pig because of its disgusting dietary habits. When the larva infest the pig's muscle and the infested pork meat (measly meat) is poorly cooked and ingested by man, the larva then completes its development into an adult tapeworm in the human intestine. The human with the adult tapeworm is then considered the definitive host.

Because of the mode of transmission of the egg and the larva of the pork tapeworm it may be advisable to eat only meats that are well cooked, refrain from eating salads, and eat fruits that can be peeled before eating. Hand washing is of utmost importance to avoid transmitting the eggs. This will not guarantee that one will not become either the intermediate or definitive host of the *Taenia solium* parasite but may reduce one's likelihood of infestation. If one does become infested the medications most commonly used are Biltricide and Albendazole. These are usually effective against the larval and adult stages of the organism.

- **Beef Tapeworm** *(Taeniarhynchus saginatus)*

This parasite is also known as the beef tapeworm because of its transmission to humans from ingesting the larvae from poorly cooked beef. This tapeworm averages fifteen to thirty feet (five to ten meters) in length. This tapeworm is more common in man than is the pork tapeworm. Treatment and prevention are the same as for the pork tapeworm.

Phylum Protozoa

There are a great number of protozoan parasites that have great importance to human disease. The most common are within the Order Dinoflagellida, the flagellates. These microscopic parasites possess a whip-like structure that aids in their locomotion. They are abundant in all oceans. Some live in the gut of crustaceans, such as the Blastdinium, while others such as the Mastiginia live in the intestines of frogs. Many use insects as the vector for human infestation. These protozoa include Malaria, Trypanosoma, Leptomonas, Leishmania, and Giardia. Toxoplasma is a protozoan usually contracted from cats or birds. Others are sexually transmitted from one infected individual to another such as Trichomonas.

Most of these parasites have a global distribution but are most abundant in warm geographical areas such as Mexico, Central and South America, and the Caribbean. The best protection from these is to avoid and take precautions against their vector. The logical steps are to use insect repellent and careful judgement on the consumption of exotic foods that may be poorly prepared and cooked. If one does come down with any symptoms (of which there may be many depending on the infestation), medical attention should be sought immediately. There are a number of medications effective against these parasites and should be initiated as soon as possible under medical supervision. Areas that are known to be endemic for malaria may cause a traveler to elect to take antimalarial drugs during their trip. Consultation with an infectious disease specialist prior to travel may be wise to determine whether a medication should be taken, and if so, which one. There are strains of malaria that have different resistance patterns to anti-malarial drugs within certain geographical areas.

•Amoebas

The Genus Entamoeba is another member of the protozoan phylum. These are commonly known as amoebas. The species within this group that affect humans are *E. coli, E. hartmanni, E. gingivalis, E. histolytica, Endolimax nana, Iodamoeba butsechlii,* and *Dientamoeba fragilis.* Most amoebas are not pathogenic but *E. histolytica* does cause one of the most serious parasitic diseases (amebiasis) in tropical and temperate countries. About 600 million people are infected with this strain although only a small fraction have symptoms. It is estimated that in some tropical countries over 40% of the population may be infected. The infection may involve not only the intestine but may also cause serious liver amebic abscesses.

Poor sanitary conditions, infected food handlers, improper disposal of sewage, or flies may be modes of disease transmission by contamination of food, water, or eating utensils. A traveler may decide to drink only bottled water or beverages and avoid ice in their drink. Avoid salads or foods that are rinsed with tap water and not cooked. Use of plastic wrapped, disposable eating utensils would be the safest alternative. Use of bottled water for brushing teeth is also advised.

Flagyl is a safe and very effective oral amebicide that reaches all body tissues. There are other agents that are also effective for specific circumstances such as Protostat and Aralen, but all should be used under proper medical supervision. Anti-malarial agents frequently used are Fansidar, Plaquenil, Daraprim, and Aralen. Daraprim and Sulfadiazine are an effective combination against toxoplasmosis.

Phylum Nematoda

The roundworms are a group of parasites that have significant importance to humans and many other animals due to their tremendous success as parasites. These parasites either invade the host through the skin or are introduced from an insect vector.

•Threadworm (Strongylida)

These parasites are known as the threadworms and are found in tropical locations. The larvae are found in the soil and penetrate the skin of individuals walking barefoot.

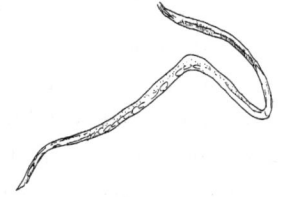

Figure 96 Threadworm

The larvae migrate to the lungs through the bloodstream and burrow their way into the air spaces in the lung. They then climb up to the back of the throat where the unsuspecting person then swallows them. The adult worm lives in the intestine laying hundreds of eggs. These eggs can hatch and reinfect the same individual or be passed out with the feces where the larva hatch and await another barefoot victim. (See Figure 96)

Protection from these is straightforward: wear shoes. Mintezol is an effective medication for these infestations.

• **Hookworm (Ancylostoma)**

This hookworm causes "creeping eruptions." These larvae penetrate the skin of individuals walking barefoot on the beach that has been littered with dog or cat feces. The larva develops into the adult hookworm that stays beneath the skin and migrates about an inch (one to two cm) a day while it eats. The parasite causes intense irritation and itching.

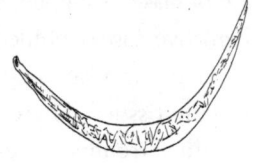

Figure 97 Hookworm

Wearing foot protection and not lying on the beach will prevent infection. Treatment is with Thiabendazole. (See Figure 97)

• **Roundworm (Ascaris)**

This large roundworm (15 to 30 cm) is most abundant in the tropics, in areas where sanitation is poor. Ascaris is common worldwide but most common in warm areas and the Orient. At one time one in every four people in the world was infested! In some geographical areas of the Orient the infestation rate is 100%. Transmission is by contamination of food and drink with the eggs. Female Ascaris can lay up to 200,000 eggs a day. Humans have been documented as having up to 1,488 worms at one time. The incredibly large number of eggs released by infested individuals makes the risk of transmission from proximity to an infected individual quite high if there are less than optimal hygiene habits.

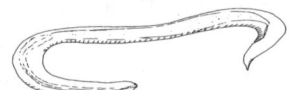

Figure 98 Roundworm

Effective treatment is available with Antiminth, Mintezol, and Vermox. (See Figure 98)

•Pinworm (Enterobiasis)

Also known as pinworms, this is a disease mainly of children but can affect individuals of all ages. This infestation is not just limited to rural areas, and is quite common in urban and suburban areas as well. The parasite resides in the large colon and migrates to the anal opening at night to release its eggs. The most common symptom is pruritis ani (itchy anus) at night. The eggs are dispersed on the person's clothing, bedding, hands, and bottom, or even on the dust of the room. Transmission can occur from inhaling contaminated air, eating without hand washing, or eating contaminated food or drink.

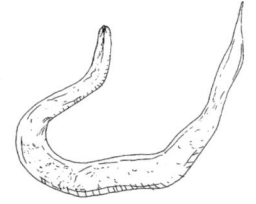

Figure 99 Pinworm

Prevention is by frequently laundering bedding and clothing, removing dust, and good personal hygiene. The medications most commonly used to eradicate the infestation are Antiminth, Mintezol, and Vermox. (See Figure 99.)

•Whipworm (Trichuriasis)

Whipworms are found worldwide, especially in tropical and subtropical areas. The same species that affect humans also affect monkeys and pigs. It only causes disease and symptoms in individuals with a heavy parasitic burden. The worm lives in the intestine and the eggs are produced and released in the feces. Transmission is by contamination of food and drink as well as poor hygiene by food handlers and nurses.

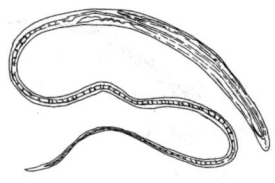

Figure 100 Whipworm

Prevention is by assuring proper hygiene and eating at establishments that require proper hygiene by their chefs and food servers. Treatment is with the use of Mintezol and Vermox. (See Figure 100)

Microbial Diseases

Microscopic organisms are ubiquitous and important for survival of all living things. These organisms are single-celled life forms and can be divided into groups that differentiate them according to their reproductive mechanisms and chemical make-up. Bacteria, yeast, fungi, mycobacteria, viruses, and prions are the major types of microbes. Many such microbial organisms are pathogenic (cause disease) to humans. Exposure to and infection by these organisms may occur in a variety of ways. Certain pathogenic strains may have specific geological niches or are endemic in certain climates. The divers' affinity to water and their search for pristine dive sites often leads to remote areas that may be cesspools of disease.

The variety of infectious agents is too numerous to cover in this text. The following is a limited list of those organisms that may pose the biggest risk at the time of preparation to the traveler.

Cholera

Cholera is caused by the organism *Vibrio cholerae*. This disease is endemic mainly in the common delta of the Ganges and Brahmaputra Rivers for the past 200 years and in the Philippines. Sporadic outbreaks have occurred in London, North America, Indonesia, Guam, Western Europe, Spain, Canada, Japan, Italy, Syria, and in several Central and Western African areas.

Transmission is mainly by water. Poor sanitary conditions with contamination of the water source are responsible for many outbreaks. The food supply is the second most common cause of dissemination of the disease to the public. The disease may cause mild or no symptoms and these carriers play a major role in the spread of the disease from one region to another. This disease affects children predominantly during pandemics. The incubation period is between six hours and twelve days. Symptoms are abrupt, watery, frequent diarrhea. The volume of the water loss from the effect of the cholera toxin on the intestinal wall frequently requires hospitalization for intravenous water replacement. Shock from severe water loss and the associated imbalances of the serum electrolytes are the most common causes of death from this disease.

Proper hygiene and the consumption of bottled water when abroad are advised in endemic areas. Avoidance of ice in beverages and food that has been rinsed is recommended. Immunization against the disease offers three to six months of protection for 60 to 80% of recipients. Many adults and children may be able to replace large volumes of fluids by mouth and endure the length of the symptoms. Carefully monitoring the balance of fluid intake and output is key to successful management. Maintaining proper hydration with fluid intake is crucial until medical help is obtained. Taking tetracycline is recommended to shorten the duration of the symptoms and to eradicate the disease from the system to avoid becoming a carrier.

Creutzfeldt Jakob Disease

This disease has assumed the common name of "Mad Cow Disease." It is caused by viral-like particles called prions and is transmitted by direct tissue contamination and via the food supply. This disease has acquired media attention recently because of the spread of the disease by pork and beef in Europe and England. The disease has a worldwide distribution. The disease rapidly spreads to the brain of the individual who progresses from good health to complete helplessness or death within one year. Incoordination, progressive dementia, myoclonus, and muscle wasting is encountered as the disease progresses. Definitive diagnosis is by brain biopsy in suspected individuals.

Avoiding pork and beef in regions known to harbor the disease is the best form of protection from this incurable and lethal disease.

Salmonella

Typhoid fever is caused by *Salmonella typhi*. Typhoid causes large-scale epidemics on a regular basis throughout the world. Water sources and food supply are the main routes of spread of the disease. Mexico had an epidemic due to spread associated with bottled beverages. *S. typhi* is an organism that lives only in humans. The bacteria is extremely hardy and can survive for prolonged periods in food and water. This will also apply to snorkels, regulators, and BCD hoses.

The bacteria are ingested and rapidly penetrate the intestinal wall and spread throughout the blood stream to all organs of the body. Symptoms include fever, abdominal pain, diarrhea, cough, a diffuse rash, headache, disorientation, profound fatigue, anemia, and pneumonia. Relapses are common after treatment. Some individuals become carriers despite resolution of symptoms. 50% of individuals after six weeks are still shedding organisms with their feces.

Other strains of Salmonella are quite common in domestic and wild animals. These infections in humans cause intestinal infections for the most part and cause diarrhea. Chills, fever, and prolonged illness may be associated with these infections.

Prevention is by the use of careful hygiene and bottled water. Recalls of prepared foods or packaged meats that cause outbreaks are heard in the media from time to time. In this sense the media is an important tool to advise and protect the public. Multiple antibiotics are effective against Salmonella although antibiotic resistance patterns are changing.

Shigella

Shigellosis is an intestinal infection in humans that is initially associated with fever and progresses to severe dysentery accompanied by abdominal cramps and at times bloody frequent stools. Several species of this bacteria are encountered in North America, Western Europe, Central America, and Japan. The incidence peaks during late summer and early fall in the United States. The bacteria survive long periods of time in water and food and can be transmitted from one person to another. Crowded living conditions, poor housing, improper sewage disposal, and contaminated water supply are associated with outbreaks of this disease.

Symptoms include bloody stools, severe abdominal cramps, anorexia, and may include fever. Children often have more devastating symptoms that include delirium, convulsions, headache, nuchal (neck) rigidity, and lethargy.

Prevention is by proper hygiene and avoidance of contaminated water and food. Identification of infected individuals and eliminating them from food handling is paramount to contain outbreaks. Treatment is directed at correcting the fluid loss, pain management, and antibiotic therapy. Ampicillin is one of the more common antibiotics used. Resistance patterns will dictate therapy and alternative antibiotics may be indicated.

Tuberculosis

Mainly two types of microorganisms, *Mycobacterium tuberculosis* and *Mycobacterium bovis* cause tuberculosis (TB). Infection is almost always by inhalation of what is called "droplet nuclei." These droplet nuclei are released into the air when an individual with "Cavitary tuberculosis" in the lungs coughs and the infective nuclei are aerosolized. These droplet nuclei can remain suspended for a prolonged period and inhaled by an unsuspecting passerby. The infection begins in the lungs and is spread throughout the body through the blood stream. An individual may harbor the infection for many months without knowing he or she is infected and spread the disease unknowingly.

TB became an epidemic during the industrial revolution due to overcrowding of urban areas. It then made a decline with improved sanitation, identification and isolation of infected individuals, then finally with the development of anti-tuberculous drugs.

Unfortunately, TB has made a comeback due to TB strains that are resistant to drugs, a significant increase in individuals with compromised immune systems (i.e., AIDS), and the increase of global transportation to areas where the disease is prevalent. Alcoholics, prisons, and Indian reservations are populations in developed countries where the disease is most prevalent. TB is found worldwide and is most common in underdeveloped countries or regions that are poverty stricken with poor healthcare delivery services.

Prevention of acquiring TB is by astute attention to those around you. Stay away from crowded areas, especially where individuals are noted to have a productive, persistent cough. If someone in the vicinity is noted to be coughing but has no other symptoms of a cold, it is best to stay away. Avoiding enclosed areas with such an individual is wise. Since these droplet nuclei can travel quite a few feet and remain aerosolized for a prolonged period, one may elect to avoid loitering in bars, restaurants, or other crowded establishments where TB in known to be endemic. Although not well studied, using a snorkel, regulator, or BCD that may have been used by an individual with TB may pose a health risk. It may be wise to buy or bring one's own equipment rather than renting in a region known to be endemic for TB. There is a vaccine also available (BCG vaccine). These vaccines have had fairly good success.

Treatment of TB is a very long process. Multiple anti-TB drugs are usually prescribed for one year or longer. Even after full treatment, an individual who has had TB could have a recurrence of the disease if in a state of poor nutrition or compromised immune status. The tuberculin test is a preparation of purified protein derivative injected just under the skin to see if an individual has an immune reaction to the test. If so, the person either has TB or has been exposed to it in the past. Medical attention and evaluation will determine whether they should be treated for an infection. If the individual has had the BCG vaccine, their tuberculin test will convert to positive, thus eliminating the benefit of this test for early infection.

Tinea Cruris and Tinea Pedis

When individuals wear wet clothing or trunks for prolonged periods with maceration of the skin, plaques and nodules may appear that are associated with development of a fungal infection. The infection is named after the anatomical area affected, cruris indicating the groin area and pedis signifying the feet, and so on. The infection is usually within a skin fold or area that is covered and maintained warm and moist for an extended period of time. Divers may be at risk from wearing wet swimwear or protective suits for prolonged time periods during a multiple dive day. Yeast infections mimic these fungal infections except that the rash is frequently a brighter red. Diabetics are at higher risk of acquiring these conditions. Hands can also be affected if wet dive gloves are continuously worn.

Prevention of this common skin condition is by changing into dry clothing soon after diving or swimming, and during surface intervals between same day dives. Removing wet footwear and allowing the feet to dry thoroughly is also recommended. Proper hygiene and the use of drying and medicated powders are usually effective treatments that can be used between dives. Systemic medication may be required in advanced cases.

Hepatitis

There are several strains of the hepatitis virus. The strain that is most important for travelers is the hepatitis A strain. This viral strain is transmitted via the fecal-oral route. An infected individual with an active case of hepatitis passes the viruses in the stool and poor hygiene may allow contamination of food or water that is then consumed by others. Individuals without prior exposure to the hepatitis A virus are at particular risk when traveling to areas where the virus is endemic with poor sanitation. The virus may also affect primates where humans may be infected from proximity to primates in endemic areas. Shellfish residing in contaminated seawater tend to concentrate the virus and human infection is known to occur from ingestion of raw or steamed shellfish dishes.

Hepatitis B is usually transmitted via transfusions of blood or blood products. Mosquitoes and bedbugs have been found to harbor the hepatitis B virus. Although not well documented to cause disease in humans, these insects may possibly transmit hepatitis B from one infected individual to another.

Fever, shaking chills, weakness, loss of appetite, right upper abdominal pain, joint pain, diarrhea, and body rash are frequent early symptoms. Dark colored urine and a yellowish tint to the skin and the whites of the eyes are seen during the icteric phase of the disease. An infected individual may have bouts of relapses after what appears to be a good recovery. A serum test will confirm the diagnosis and hospitalization and rest are important to recovery and treatment.

Prevention is by knowledge of the endemic nature of the virus to assure caution by the traveler. Proper hygiene and avoidance of shellfish in endemic areas is important. Bottled water and avoiding uncooked foods may also decrease the likelihood of ingesting contaminated food. The use of insect repellents is also recommended in endemic tropical areas.

There are immunizations available for both hepatitis A and B. The hepatitis A immunization should be administered within two weeks of hepatitis exposure. This will reduce or eliminate the severity of the symptoms. Exposure to the virus will then confer active immunity to the individual. For those exposed to primates on an ongoing basis it is recommended that immunizations be administered every four months. Immunization for hepatitis B is not recommended for travelers as it is for hospital staff.

Dengue

This illness is caused by a virus that is transmitted to humans strictly by the mosquito. The mosquito itself becomes infected when it feeds off an infected person. After eight to twelve days the mosquito becomes infective and remains so the rest of its life. The virus is transmitted into their blood stream when a mosquito feeds upon a person. There is a five to six day incubation period in the human and a febrile illness begins. Malaise, prostration, muscle and joint pain, headache, severe eye pain, and a diffuse rash are associated with the disease.

The infection is self-limiting and not life-threatening. Prevention is by using insect repellent. There is no specific treatment available. Symptomatic treatment with analgesics and rest is recommended.

Staphylococcus

There are several species of the Staphylococcus bacteria. They are among the most ubiquitous bacteria on human skin. They usually colonize the skin without causing disease but given the opportunity they will take advantage of breaks in the skin to set up an infection. Staph is the most common infection of the skin. It is the primary cause of furuncles (pimples) and folliculitis (hair follicle infections). Carbuncles are larger infections that are usually deeper into the tissues. Given the opportunity Staph can gain access to the blood stream and cause infection of any and all other tissues and organs of the body. Rashes as well as fungal and yeast infections that cause itching can lead to secondary Staph infections, especially when skin breakdown occurs from repeated scratching.

Staph produces a suppurative (pus-producing) infection. The bacteria can produce a variety of toxins that can cause destruction of blood cells (hemolytic), destruction of tissues (necrotizing), destruction of white blood cells (leukocidal), constriction of blood vessels (vasospastic), and a host of other substances that can complicate the infection. Many of these other substances can lead to severe symptoms or death. Some of these substances are lysozyme, catalase, enterotoxin, epidermolysin, fibrinolysin, hyaluronidase, lipase, thermonuclease, beta-lactamase, protease, and coagulase as well as others. The importance of these toxins is in their ability to produce severe symptoms and tissue damage that may persist beyond the treatment of the infection.

Abrasions, cuts, puncture wounds, burns, and devitalized skin are frequently secondarily infected by Staph. Diabetics and those with immune deficiencies are at particular risk of infection. Proper care of any break in the skin is of utmost importance to prevent infection from taking hold and progressing. Cleaning an injured area with antiseptic, applying an antibiotic cream or ointment, and applying a sterile dressing is the best formula to follow in the field. If redness, swelling, drainage, and pain increase, it is likely that the wound is becoming infected. Medical attention may be considered to debride and treat the wound.

Lost or Stolen Credit Cards or Money

Becoming familiar with the foreign currency and the latest exchange rate is wise for all travelers. In many locations U.S. currency is welcome and no currency exchange is necessary. It is frequently advised to bring little cash and use credit cards as often as possible. Have the merchants place the charge in the local currency on the credit card and allow your bank to convert the currency for you. This practice will assure the best possible exchange rate with no exchange fees. If spouses are traveling together it may be best to take different credit cards. For instance, one can take Visa™ and MasterCard™ while the other takes American Express™ and Discover™. In the event one loses one's cards or has them stolen requiring them to be cancelled immediately, the other person will have different cards that will not be cancelled. The currency that is brought along is best planned in the form of some cash and the rest in traveler's checks. Stolen traveler's checks may be replaced whereas cash cannot. Keeping the traveler's check receipts in a safe deposit box at the hotel will safeguard them for replacement of the traveler's checks. Many locations have ATMs that allow a traveler to obtain cash with the use of credit cards. This minimizes the amount of cash an individual will have on hand and lower the risk of losing it or having it stolen. Smaller amounts of cash can be obtained during the trip rather than having a large sum at hand during the vacation.

When going on a boat excursion there is rarely a need to purchase anything onboard. When brought aboard, the wallet or purse is only at risk of falling overboard or being stolen. It is recommended to leave all valuables in the room safe or safe deposit box at the hotel. The only cash that is usually needed on a boat dive is the tip for the crew and Divemaster.

Travelers should not carry all their cash around on their person. They should take only what they feel they will need that day, leaving the rest in the safe deposit box in the hotel. Items left in a safe deposit box may be safer than in an alternative location but not completely safe. A detailed list of the items and the amount of cash left should be made and kept on one's person or in another safe place in case of theft from the safe deposit box. It may be wise to carry only one or two credit cards at a time leaving the rest of the cards in the safe for use only if the others are lost or stolen. If credit cards are lost or stolen they are to be reported immediately. Some banks will arrange for immediate replacement and delivery to the traveler's hotel within two days.

Assaults

Assaults and robberies of travelers are common but many times avoidable if precautions are followed. Victims are fortunate if a robbery ends without physical harm. There are recommendations that can be followed to improve the likelihood of avoiding bodily harm during this most unfortunate of events that spoil a trip.

Everyone knows that when you travel all your money is on your person. The question is, where? Carrying a purse or wallet makes the target easier for a thief. Cash is the most desirable target a thief aims for. Other important documents, jewelry, laptops, and credit cards can be objects worthy of theft as well. Thieves may try to separate you from your valuables by pick-pocketing you, holding you up, or breaking into your room. There are certain times that make a traveler more vulnerable than others. We will review these and recommend solutions to decrease the vulnerability of the traveling diver.

It is a good idea to carry only what is needed on a day-to-day basis. Take only enough cash for that day and leave the rest in the hotel safe. If the day will be spent on a dive boat, bring only enough to tip the crew. It is unlikely that you will need any other money on the boat. Never pull out a large roll of money. If you are carrying a large sum of money, always separate a small amount in small bills for paying for small items. Bring along one or two credit cards if needed. Leave the rest of the cards in the safe. If with a spouse, you carry one card and let them carry a different card. It is recommended to have gratuities ready for porters and doormen.

There are several strategies and products that can make pick-pocketing much more difficult. If a woman does carry a purse she should carry one with a strong strap. Placing the strap around the neck and holding the purse firmly under the arm will deter most "grab and run" thieves. Wear your purse on the side away from the street, and on escalators on the side away from the opposite ramp. They will always try for the easiest victims. If the woman wears a blazer, coat, or jacket, placing the purse around the neck and under the arm beneath the coat will further discourage a thief, if they see the purse at all. A man may elect to carry his wallet in the front pocket during travel to discourage a rear pocket "bump and pick pocket" thief. One last strategy is to have a "decoy wallet." Keep a few singles in there and possibly expired credit cards while keeping "real" cards and currency in a hidden wallet.

Products that are available as an alternative to purses or wallets come in a variety of styles. The neck/shoulder security pouch is used much like the purse with a strong strap as described above. The fanny pack is another alternative that can be worn under one's clothing or in plain view. Both of these products may have the strap cut by a thief and taken away, although some have a steel braided cable sewn into the strap. The calf or ankle wallet wraps around the calf or ankle out of view. It will hold much less than the other pouches but remains hidden. The traveler needs to be sure that the needed cash for travel is in their pocket to maintain the wallet hidden. The hidden pocket wallet attaches to a pant loop or belt and hangs inside the pants. This is a very effective way to deter any pickpocket. Belts with zippered compartments in the back are another alternative to prevent a pickpocket from robbing you.

Environments that are conducive to thieves need to be recognized and avoided. Most robberies on the street are between sundown and sunrise. Remote, dark, abandoned areas need to be avoided at any time of day. On the other hand, very crowded locations are a pickpocket's favorite place. Escalators, boarding areas, and entrances are common locations for pickpocket strikes. Walking slowly as when window-shopping makes you an easier target, so walk quickly. Be suspicious of anyone who bumps or gets caught on something of yours. Anyone who falls or slips ahead of you may just be a decoy to slow you down so another can bump into you. Be cautious with anyone who approaches you to offer or ask anything, especially if they speak good English in a foreign land. Be aware of who is around you, and if you notice the same person in your vicinity for an extended period of time or in more than one location, be very suspicious and cautious.

Personal appearance can do much to reduce the probability of being targeted for a robbery or pickpocket. Dress casually, like the locals if possible. Carrying a camera is a dead giveaway that you are a tourist. Leave jewelry at home, including watches and wedding rings. Don't travel alone in strange places. Walk with confidence, and don't give the appearance of being lost even if you are. Never carry a weapon in a foreign country. It may get you in legal trouble and it could be used against you if you are attacked. If you think you are being followed quickly enter a well-populated area or establishment. If a car seems to be following you, turn around and walk in the opposite direction.

Travelers at the airport are recommended to stay in a group. Place bags in the middle of the group, not outside the circle. Keep all bags close and lock all suitcases. Use covered luggage tags and write the address of one's office rather than one's home. If going to the restroom, bring all your belongings or leave them with the rest of the group to watch. Have a companion escort you and use the corner stall. Do not place bags on the floor of the stall where someone could reach under the partition to grab them and run. If traveling with multiple bags and someone grabs one of them and runs, do not run after them leaving several other bags behind. A second thief will certainly carry the others away. Yell and point at the thief and hope that the authorities will spot them and detain them. Better to lose one bag and not all of them.

If you were pick-pocketed after something unusual occurred in front of you (i.e,. fall, slip, etc.), don't try to chase the thief.

Inconspicuously follow the individual that perpetrated the diversion for the thief. Get the attention of the authorities and identify the accomplice for them. They will likely lead to the pickpocket. The decoy for the thief is commonly a child or woman.

If you are involved in a robbery, do not resist. Give them what they want. This will lessen the likelihood of getting hurt and expedite the termination of the event. Thieves are interested in valuables, not in hurting you. If you have a hidden wallet you do not need to reveal it. Give them what you have in your pockets but don't resist if they attempt to search you. Do not attempt to disarm them or fight them, even if you think you may have an advantage. Do not make any sudden moves that may startle the perpetrator. Move slowly and deliberately. Do not try to call a perpetrator's bluff if they threaten to hurt you if you don't cooperate or if they claim to have a concealed weapon. Take note of their clothing and physical features and notify the authorities as soon as possible.

When staying at a hotel be sure the receptionist does not announce your room number out loud. Have them write it on your papers. The key should not have the room number on it in case it is pick-pocketed or lost. Ask for a room near the elevators and away from construction or the emergency stairwells. Ask for receipts if asked to pay in advance. Double lock the doors of your room when you are there and lock all available locking devices on the door. You may consider locking any sliding doors to a balcony or terrace and doors between suites. Lock unneeded valuables in the room safe or (even better) place them in the lobby safe deposit box. If the safe is in your room and a burglar forces his way in he could ask you to open your safe. It would be very unlikely for them to follow you down to the lobby to get items out of the safe deposit box. Cover expensive garments under other clothing on hangers. If someone knocks on the door, look through the peephole first. If you don't recognize who is there don't open it. If you didn't ask or call for anything, don't open the door. You may call and confirm with the hotel the identity of whoever the person states they may be before opening the door.

When you leave your room don't hang the "Clean my room" sign. This only announces that you are not there. It is recommended to call house keeping to tell them when to clean your room. Leaving the "Do not disturb" sign on the door gives the impression you are there. Leave the night table radio or TV set on. Leave a light on in the room for when you return. When returning to your room, always have your key ready to open the door. Do not open your door if someone is behind you or in the immediate vicinity. Walk past your room or turn to the elevator or exit. If your room door is open, don't enter. Call security and have them investigate.

Motor Vehicle Precautions

Driving an automobile in a foreign country can be tricky and may take some getting used to. The driver should obtain a list of the traffic signs and familiarize themselves with them. Driving on the opposite side of the road takes constant attention, especially when making turns at intersections. Driving on the opposite side of the car may make the driver uneasy until he or she becomes accustomed to it. A pedestrian crossing the road may be at risk of injury if they look the wrong way for oncoming traffic.

Travelers who rent automobiles should obtain the insurance offered since most drivers' primary insurance will either not cover or have very limited coverage. Obtaining a full set of maps in English for the required destinations is important. Having the routes highlighted in advance will save time and prevent losing one's way. It is also a good idea to have the phone numbers of the hotel or resort available in case one is delayed or lost. The resort personnel may be able to give advice on reaching the location.

Don't leave valuables in the car in plain view, or leave your luggage visible in the back seat, car top, or trunk. Have your key ready when approaching your car. Look inside at the front and back seat before you get in. Look around the area before getting out of the car. If in doubt, drive on and don't get out. Drive and park in well-lit and populated areas. Avoid parking near areas where someone may be hiding such as forests, garbage cans, dumpsters, alleys, etc.

When traveling with scuba tanks, the diver should store the tanks in the trunk or an area where no passengers are seated. Bumps, turns, hills, and collisions may cause severe injuries if a passenger is near a pile of tanks. The tanks in the trunk need to be secured with tank stabilizers or objects tightly packed around the tanks to keep them wedged and prevent shifting or rolling. Laying the tanks side to side may improve safety during rear-end collisions if the valve is broken off and the tank or valve becomes a missile.

Know where you are going to avoid getting lost in the "wrong" neighborhood. Always keep the doors locked and consider keeping the windows closed if anyone is near the vehicle. If lost, drive at the normal speed to avoid attracting attention. Don't stop to make a call in the "wrong" neighborhood. Drive in the lane furthest from the sidewalk and keep enough distance from the car ahead to always be able to drive around them and get away. Avoid driving at night especially when alone.

If you encounter a disabled car with a stranded driver, do not get out of your car to assist them. You may let them know you will call for help. Do not open your door or window for anyone who approaches the car to ask for directions or offering to give or sell something to you. Be very suspicious of anyone attempting to get your attention and pointing at the car as if something is wrong. Do not stop. Proceed to the nearest gas station to inspect the car.

It is highly recommended that you not hitchhike either

locally or in a foreign country. You are at the mercy of whoever picks you up. Likewise, do not pick up hitchhikers no matter how friendly or beautiful they may look. Do not accept rides from strangers offering a ride. If you use a taxi, only use marked taxi cars. Exit a taxi only when you are sure you are at your destination and after you have received your correct change.

Auto accidents can be an event that can lead to injury, assault, or carjacking. Most carjackings involve pedestrians or minor car accidents. The thieves try to damage the car as little as possible. The "bump and rob" scenario is a frequent ploy to get you to stop and get you out of the car. There is always more than one individual in the thieves' car and does not only occur in remote areas. A high level of suspicion is important. If you think a "bump and rob" scenario may be unfolding don't get out of the car. Signal or tell the occupants of the other car to follow you. Remember the license plate number and the type of car as you drive off to a service station or police station. When you get out of the car lock the door, take the key, and enter the service station or police station and have someone else come out with you to inspect the damage.

If you are a victim of a carjacking and are approached by an armed assailant, don't resist. Let them have the car and get out of the area. Take note of the thieves' clothing, physical features, and the plates and type of auto they were in. Report the incident to the authorities immediately.

Imprisonment

There are many reasons a traveler may get arrested. Engaging in illegal activities, attempting to smuggle illegal goods, becoming involved in altercations, and not cooperating with authorities are the most frequent. Being accused of espionage, being involved in anti-government propaganda, and aiding and abetting criminals are not as common but in certain political and geographical areas care must be taken to not have one's actions misinterpreted by local officials.

If you are arrested, do not resist. Resisting arrest may lead to much more serious charges or physical harm. Cooperate with the authorities. If you have nothing to hide, cooperate fully with police and you may be found to have been detained without cause. If on the other hand you have been caught involved in illegal activities or you are still detained despite not having done anything illegal, you may ask to contact the United States Consul. The U.S. Consul may not be able to get you out of prison but they can assist in obtaining a local attorney. The U.S. Consul can visit with you and ensure that your accommodations and treatment are humane. They can notify family and coordinate sending you money, food, and clothing.

Be cautious about police imposters. Thieves commonly own police uniforms and fake badges, especially in third world countries. They rarely own well-kept police vehicles. If you have not been involved in anything illegal or anything that can be remotely interpreted as illegal, be suspicious about being approached by the authorities. Robberies and carjackings can be setup by the phony police approach. Police never ask to see your money. If they do, or want to search you, ask to be taken to the police station. If in your car, show your license through the window without opening it. If they insist you get out of the car and you are suspicious of their authenticity, let them know you will follow them to the police station.

NOTES

Appendix 1

Example of Emergency Procedures Check List

EMERGENCY PROCEDURES
MYLES O' JOY

To contact Emergency Medical Services (EMS) or Rescue Services refer to the Emergency Action Plan Sheet (EAPS) on page 6. All emergency phone numbers and appropriate radio frequencies are listed on the EAPS. The ship's call numbers and all vital ship information are located on the first page of the Yacht Log also located at the cabin helm station and on the last page of this manuscript.

For life-threatening emergencies a caller is to observe the following procedure:
1) Be sure the ship to shore radio is on and set to the appropriate frequency (usually channel 16).
2) Press the transmission button on the microphone to speak.
3) Clearly and slowly repeat "Mayday" three times and identify yourself by stating the name of your vessel (Myles O' Joy) and whom you are attempting to reach (i.e., "Mayday, Mayday, Mayday, this is the Myles O' Joy requesting assistance from the U.S. Coast Guard").

4) Release the transmission button to wait for a response.
5) If no response is obtained repeat the above procedure.
6) After obtaining a response from the Rescue Personnel identify vessel name, registration #, and radio call sign in a clear, calm, concise manner (see last sheet for #'s).
7) State your location or compass heading to a known point.
8) Describe the nature of the emergency.
9) Follow the directions of the Rescue Personnel.

For Emergencies where no life is at risk a caller is to observe the following procedure:

1) Be sure the ship to shore radio is on and set to the appropriate frequency (usually channel 16).
2) Press the transmission button on the microphone to speak.
3) Clearly and slowly repeat "Security" three times and identify yourself by stating the name of the your vessel (Myles O' Joy) and whom you are attempting to reach (i.e., "Security, Security, Security, this is the Myles O' Joy requesting assistance from the U.S. Coast Guard").
4) Release the transmission button and await a response.
5) If no response is obtained repeat the above procedure.
6) After obtaining a response from the Rescue Personnel identify vessel name, registration #, and radio call # in a clear, calm, concise manner (see last sheet for #'s).
7) State location or compass heading to a known point.
8) Describe the nature of the emergency.
9) Follow the directions of the Rescue Personnel.

Injury
1) Evaluate extent and nature of injury.
2) Take appropriate measures to prevent further injury.
3) Take appropriate measures to avoid other passenger injuries.
4) Institute first aid and/or CPR as necessary (first aid procedures are found within the first aid kit in the aft-cabin along with an oxygen tank).
5) Contact the EMS if appropriate.
6) Contact the victim's "emergency contact person" if appropriate.
7) Document all aspects of the incident.

APPENDIX

Man Overboard

1) Stop or turn vessel as deemed appropriate.
2) Throw life ring to victim (located on stern railing), maintaining hold of end of life ring line.
3) When the victim grasps line, pull them in slowly and assist them aboard.
4) If the victim is disabled or unconscious, dispatch rescue personnel wearing life vest to retrieve victim.
5) Upon recovering victim evaluate them for extent and nature of injuries.
6) Warm them with blanket and institute first aid and/or CPR as necessary (first aid procedures are found within the first aid kit in the aft-cabin along with an oxygen tank).
7) Contact the EMS if appropriate.
8) Contact the victim's "emergency contact person" if appropriate.
9) Document all aspects of the incident.

Fire

1) Assess extent and type of fire (i.e., type A- cloth, wood, etc.; type B- gasoline, oil, etc.; type C- electrical; type D- flammable metal).
2) Evacuate all passengers in vicinity and have them along with the crew don their life vests (located under the bench on the flying bridge).
3) Assess extent and nature of all injuries to passengers.
4) Institute first aid and/or CPR if appropriate (first aid procedures are located in the first aid kit in the aft-cabin along with an oxygen tank).
5) Eliminate fuel to fire (i.e., types A and D- remove all flammable material from area; type B- shut off fuel lines; type C- shut off electrical circuits).
6) Use appropriate fire extinguishers to extinguish fire (located on the inside of door of the cabinet on the flying bridge, on the starboard side of the entrance to the cabin, and to the right of the refrigerator in the galley).
7) Deploy the life raft if available and appropriate.
8) Have passengers abandon ship if appropriate.
9) Contact the EMS if appropriate.

Vessel Taking Water
1) Assess location and extent of leak.
2) Have all crew and passengers don their life jackets (located under the bench on the flying bridge) and move to the upper decks.
3) Activate all bilge pumps, designate personnel to use manual pumps or buckets.
4) Use the emergency leak repair kit if appropriate (located in the cabinet on the flying bridge).
5) Shut off engine if leak from engine hose.
6) Shut off engine, close sea cock, disconnect intake water hose, place end in bilge, restart engine to act as bilge pump.
7) Deploy the life raft if available and appropriate.
8) Have passengers abandon ship if appropriate.
9) Contact the EMS if appropriate.

Vessel Collision
1) Assess extent and location of vessel damage.
2) Assess extent and nature of passenger injuries.
3) Have the crew and passengers don life vests (located under the bench on the flying bridge).
4) Designate crew and available manpower to limit further vessel damage and to attend to the injured as the circumstances would dictate.
5) Carry out a crew and passenger head count to account for all individuals aboard.
6) Attempt to contain any fires by appropriate means (fire extinguishers are located on the inside of the door of the cabinet on the flying bridge, on the starboard side of the cabin entrance, and to the right of the refrigerator in the galley).
7) Attempt to limit taking on water by appropriate means – see Vessel Taking On Water section. (Emergency leak repair kit located in the cabinet on the flying bridge.)
8) Contact the EMS.
9) Deploy the life raft if available and appropriate.
10) Have the passengers abandon ship if appropriate.

All Other Emergencies
1) Assess nature of emergency.
2) Evaluate potential for injury to passengers and crew.
3) Evaluate potential for damage to vessel.
4) Take appropriate action to limit injury or damage.
5) Evaluate need for donning life vests.
6) Contact the EMS if appropriate.
7) Evaluate need to abandon ship.

Documentation
It cannot be stressed enough to document all aspects of an emergency scenario. Memorializing the circumstances of an emergency by writing them down should be done at the time of the event (possibly by designating a scribe) or if the circumstances won't allow, as soon as possible after the situation has stabilized. If circumstances allow, photographs, audio tapes, video tapes, specimens, and salvaged items may be of benefit in memorializing the event. When documenting an emergency, inclusion of the following information is essential:

1) Date, day, and time of all events.
2) Circumstances leading up to the emergency.
3) Description of the event.
4) Aftermath of the event.
5) Individuals involved.
6) Witnesses of event.
7) Description of injuries incurred.
8) Description of damages incurred.
9) Assistance, first aid, or CPR rendered and by whom.
10) Response to aid or treatment.
11) EMS contacts and their responses.

Any and all pertinent information or descriptions.

Appendix 2

Example of Emergency Action Plan

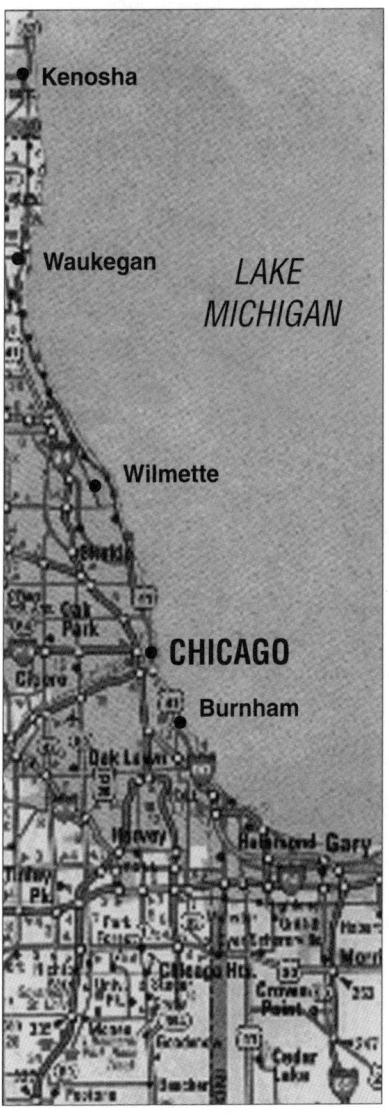

Monitored Radio Channels

Coast Guard	Ch. 9, 12, 16
Bridges	Ch. 12, 16
Harbors	Ch. 12, 16

Milwaukee/Racine Area

Mt. Pleasant Rescue	(414) 554-8822

Hyperbaric Chamber
St. Luke Hospital	(414) 649-6577

Waukegan Area

Waukegan Coast Guard	(847) 251-0185

Chicago Area

Emergency	911

Coast Guard
Calumet Harbor	(312) 353-0278
Wilmette Station	(847) 251-0185
Search & Rescue	(312) 353-0278
Air Station	(847) 657-2145
Rescue Emergency	(847) 729-6190

Chicago Marine Police	(312) 744-4817

Hyperbaric Chambers
Lutheran G. Hospital, *1775 W. Dempster, Park Ridge, IL*	(847) 696-2210
Edgewater Hospital, *5700 N. Ashland, Chicago, IL*	(773) 878-6000
St. James Hospital, *Chicago Ridge & Lincoln Highway*	(773) 756-1000
Jackson Park Hospital, *7531 S. Stoney Island, Chicago, IL*	(773) 947-7500

Harbors

Milwaukee	(414) 286-3511
Kenosha	(414) 653-4052
Waukegan	(847) 244-3133
Belmont	(312) 742-7673
Diversey	(312) 742-7762
Monroe	(312) 742-7643
Burnham	(312) 747-7009
Divers Alert Network	(919) 684-8111

Index

A

abandon ship 177, 181, 182
abandonment of the ship 187
abdominal thrust 46
  See also Heimlich maneuver
Ace wraps™ 6, 7
aground 192, 193
air 88
air embolus 49, 106
air horn 20, 120, 149, 151
airway 42, 45-47, 69, 71, 80, 111, 112
alcohol 7, 51, 60, 104, 132-134
allergic reaction 5
allergies 5, 8, 9
alligator/crocodile attacks 72
alligators 131
altered mental status 58, 79, 90
alternate air source 100
alternate second stage 130
ammonia 4, 134
amnesia 69
amoebas 224
amputation 72, 74, 147
anaphylactic shock 9, 42, 90
anaphylaxis 42, 111
anchor 16, 19, 193-195, 198-200, 202
anchor drag 119, 196, 197
anchor line 195
anchor purchase 198
anesthetic cream 5, 6
angina 87
angry seas 180
  See also heavy seas; high waves; high seas
anti-emetic 4
antibiotic cream 5, 236
antibiotic ointment 7, 47, 56, 131, 141
antihistamine 5
antiseptic 4, 236
anxiety 42, 87, 92, 98, 210
aorta 82
arrest 206, 244, 245
  See also imprisonment
artery 49, 50, 74, 75, 79, 85, 86
artificial airway 47, 48
artificial ventilations 47
aspiration 4, 33, 50, 58, 66, 71, 76, 77, 138, 147, 158, 187
aspirin 4, 81, 87, 88, 209
assault 83, 84, 205, 238
attacks 97, 131, 133, 135, 137-140

B

bandages 6, 7
barotrauma 103-105, 111
  See also lung expansion injury; decompression injury
barracuda 72, 140
basilar skull fracture 62, 63
Battle sign 62
BCD 23, 100, 111, 112, 114, 115, 123-126, 144, 153-155, 158, 230, 232
  See also bouyancy compensation device
bedbugs 216, 217
beef tapeworm 223
belt 20
Betadine™ 4, 7, 51
binoculars 15, 22
blackflies 219
bleed 81, 83
bleeding 6-10, 31, 33, 35, 39, 49, 51, 52, 57, 62-64, 68-76, 78-82, 84, 85, 88, 105, 137, 140
  See also hemorrhage and blood loss

bleeding site 74
blister 52
blistering 52
blistering reactions 6
blood 74
blood circulation 32, 49, 79, 92
blood flow 6, 33, 35, 69, 86, 90
blood loss 42, 52, 72, 74, 76, 79, 89, 138, 147
  See also bleeding and hemorrhage
blood lost 76
blood pressure 9, 28-31, 64, 79, 88, 89, 91, 92, 135
blood pressure monitors 30
blood vessel 5, 68, 73, 76, 80, 81, 85, 88-90, 92, 135
blunt injury 62, 63, 146
boots 20
bradycardia 58
brain 34, 35, 37-40, 49, 59, 60, 64, 69, 70, 83, 84, 88-90, 109, 138, 229
brain injuries 62
breathe 100, 115
breathing 44, 50, 55, 64, 69, 70, 78, 80, 98, 99, 134, 135
bristle worms 134
buddy breathing 122
buddy line 116
buddy separation 115, 116
  See also separation
bump and rob 244
buoy 12-14, 18, 22, 113
buoyancy compensation device 20
  See also BCD
Bureau of Consular Affairs 205
burglary 206
burn 5-7, 52-57, 89, 171, 236
burn cream 5-7, 55
burn victim 54

C

call back signal 202
call-back 146
capillary refill 33
capsized vessel 203, 204
carbon dioxide 115
carbon monoxide 107, 108
carbon monoxide detector 16
carbon monoxide sensors 23, 108
cardiac 171
cardiac arrest 57, 85

cardiac contusion 78
cardiogenic shock 87, 91
carjacking 244, 245
carotid arteries 6, 64
carotid pulse 30
carotid sinus syndrome 111
cash 236-239
cast 6
  See also splints
cerebellar function 40
cerebrospinal fluid 62, 63
cerebrospinal fluid leakage 63
cervical cord injury 38
cervical fracture 69
cervical spine 38
cervical spine (neck) injury 40, 80
chemical burns 55
chemicals 133
chest compressions 43, 44
chest thrusts 47
choke 76, 77, 143
cholera 228
circulate 42
circulation 32, 33, 50, 68, 69, 78, 90, 91, 106, 133, 138, 208
Coast Guard viii, 1, 12, 93, 177, 180, 181
cold 97
collapsed lung 29
  See also pneumothorax
collision 2, 180, 181
coma 63, 69, 80, 88, 108
  See also unconscious
comatose 59, 65, 111
compartment syndrome 32, 68, 86
compound or comminuted fractures 80
concussion 35, 69
  See also loss of consciousness
cone shell 131, 133
confusion 58, 59, 71, 79
  See also disorientation
conjunctiva 33
consciousness 58, 71
convulsions 60, 70, 231
  See also epileptic fits; seizure
coral 4, 131, 132
core body temperature 57, 60
core temperature 31, 58, 60
cotton balls 7
cough 4, 33, 46, 49, 76, 107, 143, 209, 210, 231, 232

INDEX

CPR (cardio-pulmonary resuscitation) 28, 41-47, 49, 57, 60, 63, 70, 78, 80, 82, 83, 85, 87, 88, 91, 92, 103, 106, 135, 138, 158, 162, 187
cradle or arm carry 161
cramps 59, 99, 230, 231
cranial nerves 36, 37
credit cards 236-239
Creutzfeldt Jakob Disease 229
cricothyroidotomy 47
crocodiles 131
crocodilians 138
crush injury 78-80, 184
crush or penetrating chest injuries 49
currency 236, 237, 239
current 13, 19, 98, 119, 133, 144, 148, 153, 169, 185, 186, 192, 193, 195, 201
current line 12, 13, 23, 145
cyanosis 33, 49

D

DAN (Divers Alert Network) 2, 27
death 37, 68, 69, 76, 86, 88, 108, 128, 131, 132, 169, 171, 206, 208, 229, 236
death rate 80
decompression illness 88, 207
decompression injuries 3, 49
  See also barotrauma; lung expansion injury
decompression sickness 3, 101, 102, 111
decongestants 104
deep vein thrombosis 208, 209
deformity 32, 56, 70, 80
dehydration 90
dengue 235
depressed skull fracture 62, 63
dewatering 191, 192
diarrhea 228, 230, 234
direct pressure 74-76, 84, 138
discoloration 33, 62, 68, 70, 79
disorientation 59, 71, 99, 105, 230
  See also confusion
dive computer 20
dive flag 12, 23, 145, 146
dive skin 20
dive table 20, 23
  See also recreational dive planner

dive wheel 23
dizziness 59, 87, 89, 108, 109, 213
Do-Si-Do tow 156
document 37, 39
documentation 35, 92-94
dragging anchor 195, 196
drift 197
drift lead 198
drowning 76

E

ear 7, 29, 33, 41, 54, 97, 103-105, 109
ecchymosis 33
eels 72
electrical burns 56
electrical current 169
electrical failure 200
electrical fires 190
electronic underwater communicator 20
emboli 88, 209
embolizing 209
embolus 209
Emergency Action Plan (EAP) 2
emergency ascent bottle 113, 128
  See also self-contained ascent bottle
emergency leak repair kit 2, 17, 177
emergency medical kit 3, 4
EMS (Emergency Medical System) viii, 1-3, 27, 93, 118, 181, 187
emergency procedures checklist 2
engine failure 199, 200
engine power 171
entanglement 18, 112-114, 121, 132, 182, 203
entrapment 112, 121
entrapped 114
epileptic fits 70
  See also convulsions and seizures
EPIRB (Emergency Position Indicating Radio Beacon) 172
equipment malfunction viii
esophagus 106
exhaustion 98
  See also fatigue
expanding circle 121
expanding square 120
explosion 54, 81, 84, 171, 187, 189
external bleeding 89
  See also hemorrhage; bleeding; blood loss

extremity fractures 68
eye 7, 9, 33, 37, 60, 62, 72, 83, 105, 129, 130, 137, 139, 235
eye injuries 4
eye shield 9

F

fat embolus 68, 81, 88
fatigue 44, 58, 77, 98, 99, 109, 114, 128, 148, 153, 155, 156, 160, 213, 230
  See also exhaustion
fear 92, 109
femoral pulse 30, 41
fever 230, 231, 234
  See also hyperthermia
finger-nose test 40
fins 20
fire 2, 55, 56, 94, 171, 172, 181, 187-192
fire burns 54
fire extinguisher 2, 17, 188
fire sponge 134
fireman's carry 161
first aid kit 2, 4, 183, 211
first degree burn 52, 54
Flag A or Alpha 23
flail chest 78
flap valve 51
flare gun 17
flares 2, 151, 172, 183
flaring out 100
flashlight 14, 16, 119
  See also lamp; light
fleas 217
float 12, 14, 15, 23
flow of blood 64
fluke worms 221
foot-shoulder tow 156
foreign bodies 8
fracture 32, 33, 39, 56, 57, 62-64, 68 69, 78, 80, 81

G

Glasgow Coma Scale 35, 36
gloves 20
GPS (Global Positioning System) 15, 171, 173, 183, 196-198
great vessels 79, 82

H

hand-pull exit 162
head count 202
head injury 33, 34, 62, 69, 70, 92
headache 59, 64, 104, 105, 108, 213, 230, 231, 235
heart 41, 42, 49, 59, 68, 71, 78, 82, 86, 87, 89-92, 103, 106
heart attack 4, 9, 86, 87, 91, 110
heart rate 9, 28-30, 42, 64, 79, 87, 108, 135
heat exhaustion 58, 59
heat loss 57, 58, 148
heat stroke 59, 91
heatstroke 58
heavy seas 195
  See also angry seas; high waves; rough water; high seas
Heimlich maneuver 45
  See also abdominal thrust
hemoptysis 49
hemorrhage 32, 73, 76, 79, 105
  See also bleeding; blood loss
hemostasis 73
hemothorax 45, 49, 78, 82
hepatitis 233
high oxygen concentrations 3
high seas 14
  See also rough water; high waves
high waves 149, 151
  See also angry seas; heavy seas; rough water; high seas
hookworm 226
horn 143
hot liquid burns 55
hydration 109
hyperthermia 9, 58, 70, 90
  See also fever
hyperventilation 98
hyphema 33
hypothermia 9, 57, 58, 98, 111, 148, 187, 204
hypovolemic shock 52, 79, 89

I

ice 5, 72, 81, 91, 132, 133, 229
imbalance 69
immobilization 64, 65
immobilize 92
impacted fracture 32

imprisonment 244
  See also arrest
incoordination 229
inferior vena cava 82
injury 2
insect repellent 25, 217, 219, 220, 224, 234, 235
insecticide 216, 220
internal bleeding 4, 32, 33, 79, 85, 86
  See also bleeding and hemorrhage
internal damage 147
intracranial bleeding 63
inverted 127
isopropyl alcohol 4

J
jellyfish 4, 131, 132
jellyfish stings 4
jet lag 213, 214
jugular veins 6

K
knife 20

L
laceration 7, 8, 70, 80, 131
ladder 13, 19, 147
lamp 14, 16, 20, 113, 118, 147
  See also light; flashlight
leech 220
level of consciousness 77
lice 216
life jacket 181, 182, 184, 186, 187, 192
life raft 15, 181, 182, 192
life ring 13, 14, 185, 187
  See also throwable ring
life vest 2, 12, 185, 187, 203
lifeboat 12
  See also raft
light 12, 149, 150
  See also lamp; flashlight
lightning 169, 170, 201, 202
lightning bolt 170
lightning protection system 170
lightning strike 170
lights 23, 172
lipoid pneumonia 106, 107

local anesthesia 5
local anesthetic 5
local pressure 85
logbooks 24
lookout 146, 181, 186
losing consciousness 79, 111, 185
loss of blood 79
loss of consciousness 69, 89, 108
  See also concussion
loss of coordination 59, 108
loss of sensation 68
  See also numbness
lost at sea 148, 171, 173
lost consciousness 69, 211
lost diver 118, 150, 151
  See also missing diver
lumbar spine 38
lumbar spine injury 40
lung expansion injuries 9
  See also barotrauma; decompression injury
lungs 89

M
magnifying glass 8
major blood vessels 105
malaria 223, 224
man overboard 2, 171, 180, 184-186, 203
marine radio 2
  See also ship to shore radio
marker buoy 14, 118, 119, 185
mask 3, 8, 9, 20, 72, 129, 143, 144, 148, 154, 159
medical kit 10
medication 4, 5
mental status 35, 38
mirror 119, 149, 172, 183
missing diver 23
  See also lost diver
mite 214, 218
Moray Eels 139
morays 131, 139
mosquito 214, 219
motor deficit 38
  See also paralysis; weakness
mouth 33
mouth to mouth resuscitation 114, 156, 159
  See also rescue breathing

mouth to mouth breathing 48
mouth-to-mouth rescue breathing 159

N

nasal decongestant 5
nausea 105, 108
near drowning 3
neck injury 63, 69, 80, 85
nematocysts 132, 133
nerve 5, 38, 50, 68, 92
nerve injury 40
nerves 65, 68, 80, 81, 85
neurogenic shock 92
neurological exam 34
neurological survey 34
nitrogen narcosis 99, 101
nose 33
numbness 32, 39, 40, 64, 65, 101, 133, 208
See also loss of sensation

O

obstructed airway 45
octopus 20, 23
orientation 70
out of air 122, 123
out-of-air 99, 100, 125
oxygen 3, 4, 30, 35, 48, 55, 70, 77, 87, 88, 90-92, 106, 108, 109, 114, 115, 188, 207, 209
oxygen by mask 103
oxygen tank 3
oxygen therapy 55, 107
oxygen toxicity 70, 108, 111
oxygenation 34

P

packstrap carry 161, 162
pain 32, 34, 39, 42, 52, 53, 64, 70, 81, 87, 101, 104, 105, 134, 141, 208, 231, 234, 236
painful 52
panic 99, 125, 128-130, 154
panic attack 210
panic diver 154, 155
paralysis 38, 64, 70, 80, 81, 88, 89, 101, 133, 134
See also motor deficit; weakness

parasites ix, 214-216, 221, 222, 224
pedal pulse 30
penetrate 82, 83
penetrating abdominal injuries 82
penetrating injury 62, 76, 81-83, 85
peripheral nerve 38
peripheral nerve injury 38
peroxide 4, 7, 51
petroleum ointment 5, 6
PFDs (Personal Flotation Device) 12
phone 2, 15, 201
pinworm 227
pneumonia 230
pneumothorax 49, 50, 78, 82, 105, 106
See also collapsed lung
pocket mask 44, 77, 158, 159
pony bottle 114
poor coordination 101, 105
pork tapeworm 222, 223
power failure 15, 171, 172, 199, 200
precordial emphysema 49
pressure point 72, 74, 75
propeller injury 72, 74, 146, 185
protozoan parasites 223
provisions 182, 183, 204
pulmonary arrest 171
pulmonary barotrauma 88, 97, 105, 106
See also lung expansion injuries; decompression injuries
pulmonary embolus 29, 208, 209
pulse 30-32, 41, 44, 49, 59, 70, 77, 79, 87
pulse rate 30
pulse rhythm 30
pulses 30, 42, 56, 68, 69, 81, 85, 89
puncture 7, 51, 70, 74, 131
puncture wounds 6, 236
pupils 37

R

raccoon sign 62
radar 15, 197
radar ranges 197
radial artery 74
radial pulse 30, 41
radio 2, 15, 183, 201, 202
radio log 15
raft 15, 16, 23, 61, 182, 183, 187, 194
See also life raft; life boat

raft off 17
rapid ascent 143
rapid respirations 49
rashes 5
recall system 118
reciprocal U-pattern 120, 121
Recreational Dive Planner 102
   See also dive table; dive wheel
reel 20, 23
regulator 20, 23, 100, 111, 113, 118, 125, 128, 154, 159, 230, 232
repetitive dives 57
rescue breath 43, 82
rescue breathing 29, 41, 42, 44, 45, 47, 49, 51, 63, 76-78, 106, 112, 134, 158-160
   See also mouth to mouth breathing
respiration 28, 29, 41, 42, 58, 71, 77, 106, 108, 111 133
respiratory arrest 80, 85
respiratory difficulty 34
respiratory distress 81
respiratory failure 106
respiratory fatigue 29
respiratory rate 29, 41, 77, 79, 99, 115
reverse squeeze 5, 104
ring sign 62
rope 8, 18, 19, 57, 75
rough water 14, 119, 184, 186, 199-201
   See also high seas; high waves; angry seas; heavy seas
rough weather 203
roundworm 225, 226
rule of nines 53

S

safe 237, 238, 241
safe deposit box 237, 241
safety bar 123
safety stop 4, 100, 102, 123, 138, 153
salmonella 230
sandflies 217
sausage buoy 14, 20, 119, 143, 149, 151, 155
scissors 8, 22
scorpionfish 131
sea anchor 12
sea snake 131, 135
sea urchin 140

search 21-23, 117-119, 121, 171, 186
search patterns 120
seasickness 60, 61
second anchor 19, 195, 198
second-degree burns 52
secondary drowning 76
seizures 57, 59, 63, 70, 71, 80, 85, 109, 110, 171
   See also epileptic fits; convulsions
self-contained ascent bottle 20, 114
   See also emergency ascent bottle
sensation 39, 85
sensory loss 39, 40
separation 115-118
   See also buddy separation
shark 131, 135, 137
shark attack 72, 74, 135, 137, 138
Shigella 230
ship to shore radio 1, 15, 172, 201
   See also marine radio
shivering 58, 98
shock 31, 53, 55, 72, 78, 80, 82, 85, 88-90, 110, 111, 138, 229
shore dives 1
shortness of breath 49, 107, 108, 209
shouts 120
sinuses 103, 105
skull 36, 37, 63, 69, 70, 83, 85
skull fracture 39, 62, 63
slate 20, 23, 24
smoke inhalation 3, 54, 55
spinal cord 36, 64
spinal cord injury 36, 38, 40, 64, 78, 92
spinal injury 34, 38, 40, 42, 62, 65, 66, 79, 92
spine 34, 38, 65, 79, 92
spine fractures 64
splint 56, 68, 69, 72
   See also cast
splinting 57, 68, 81
spread eagle 127
Staphylococcus 235
steroid cream 5-7, 132, 134
stethoscope 9
stinging sponges 134
stingrays 131
stonefish 131
straddle-tank tow 155
strenuous 86, 88
stress 86, 98, 99, 110

stresses 87
stressful 128, 130
stroke 87, 88, 110
sunburn 5, 54
superior vena cava 82
surge 119, 144, 153, 162, 192, 193
swelling 31-33, 57, 62, 68, 70, 80, 105, 134, 236

T

tailbone 65
taking on water 2, 171, 177, 181, 192, 203
tangled 112
tank 3, 20, 23, 98, 100, 113, 114, 118, 122-125, 147, 158
tank banger 20
tank-straddle 154
tank-valve tow 156
tape 7, 8
tapeworm 221-223
TB (Tuberculosis) 231
temperature 28, 31, 59, 60, 79
tenderness 32-34, 39, 56, 64, 65, 70, 208
tension pneumothorax 45, 49, 50, 78, 82, 106
thermometer 8, 9, 31
third-degree burns 52
thoracic spine injuries 78
threadworm 225
three-quarter prone position 65, 66, 71, 77
three-quarters prone position 45
throwable flotation ring 13, 14
  See also life ring
throwing up 143
  See also vomiting
tick 214, 218
Tinea Cruris 233
Tinea Pedis 233
tourniquet 6, 8, 72, 74-76, 135, 138, 141
tow 76, 154-156, 158, 159, 161, 193, 199
toxic 9, 90, 91, 108
toxic shock 90
toxicity 29, 30
toxin 5, 35, 42, 70, 89, 91, 131, 132-134, 229, 235, 236

trachea 6, 30, 41, 47, 64, 105
trapped 114
traveler's checks 237
Trendelenburg position 92
tsetse fly 217
turbulence 210-212
type A fires 188
type B fires 188, 189
type C fires 188, 190
type D fires 188, 190

U

unconscious 45, 46, 69, 97, 110, 186, 187
unconscious diver 110
unconscious victim 32
unconsciousness 35, 69, 101
  See also coma; concussion
uncooperative 35
unresponsive 35, 37, 49, 71
unresponsive drowning 77

V

vein 50, 75
vessel collisions 83
vinegar 4, 132-134
visibility 144
vital signs 9, 28, 44, 57, 60, 65, 71, 79, 81, 87, 92, 103, 106
vomit 44, 61, 65
vomiting 77, 105, 108, 109, 158
  See also throwing up

W

wallets 15
water temperature gauge 20
wave 185
waves 17, 119, 144, 162, 179, 183, 184, 186, 192, 193, 201, 203
weak 59
weakness 38, 40, 64, 70, 101, 108
  See also motor deficit; paralysis
weights 20
wet suit 20-22
whiplash injury 57
whipworm 227
whistle 16, 20, 120, 143, 149, 151